PROFESSIONAL ETHICS IN NURSING

PROFESSIONAL ETHICS IN NURSING

Edited by
Joyce E. Thompson
and
Henry O. Thompson

KRIEGER PUBLISHING COMPANY
MALABAR, FLORIDA

Original Edition 1990

Printed and Published by
ROBERT E. KRIEGER PUBLISHING CO., INC.
KRIEGER DRIVE
MALABAR, FLORIDA 32950

Library of Congress Cataloging-in-Publication Data

Professional ethics in nursing / edited by Joyce E. Thompson and Henry
    O. Thompson.
      p. cm.
   ISBN 0-89464-352-5 (alk. paper)
   1. Nursing ethics. I. Thompson, Joyce E. II. Thompson,
Henry O.
  [DNLM:1. Ethics, Nursing WY 85 P963]
RT85.P76 1990
174'.2—dc19
DNLM/DLC
for Library of Congress   89-2667
                                          CIP

10 9 8 7

CONTENTS

FOREWORD

WHY AND WHO?

There are hundreds of articles and dozens of books now available for nurses interested in studying ethics. With the knowledge explosion and all the new duties expected of them today, nurses might wonder why bother with ethics? If that question is answered positively, the next step is where to begin? We hope in this series of essays, selected from the many available and including some of the editors' own thoughts, to give a rationale and the beginnings of understanding.

The text can be used by itself or as a supplement to a standard course on ethics, for courses on issues, for professional development, for short courses during the regular curriculum, for continuing education, and for self-study. Our central concern is the professional nurse, but others may benefit from this focus on ethics in their own profession. We hope this anthology will be useful to nurses from the beginning of their education to wherever they are in their career. With that educational perspective in mind, we offer the following as learning objectives.

Objectives

1. To sensitize the nurse and other health care professionals to the role that ethics plays in the practice of one's profession.
2. To provide an overview for nurses and other health care professionals on the nature of professional ethics in the health fields.
3. To pose the moral question of whether nurses *should* study ethics and to offer some teaching strategies for those who decide to learn about ethics.
4. To explore the nature of ethical decision making for nurses and other health care professionals.
5. To explore major issues involved in nursing research and human experiments that have ethical bases.
6. To offer a resource for nurses interested in exploring the nature of professional ethics.

IN HONORIUM

Dean Claire F. Fagin
Dean Therese Stewart

IN APPRECIATION

A preface is the time of acknowledgment and disclaimer. The latter is relatively simple; the editors waive responsibility for errors of interpretation and editorial content. The former is more difficult. We offer gratitude to the authors and publishers for permission to reprint these essays. Our thanks extend beyond the printed page to the pioneering work that many have done. The ground work represented here makes it possible to talk about nursing ethics in a realistic way. Nursing ethics is gradually out of the "maybe" stage to become a real thing. It is not yet in full swing in educational curricula but the swing is in that direction. Our appreciation goes beyond our authors to those who have encouraged our work and to those who have assisted the development of this text. Then there are those who never knew us but whose work, writing, story, life has become a part of our own. They include moral philosophers and moral theologians and practitioners of the scientific art or artistic science called nursing. Among those who have known us, and who are now part of our lives, are colleagues, family, and friends gathered over the years. These are all a part of our work in progress and this work in particular.

ABBREVIATIONS

AJN	American Journal of Nursing
ANA	American Nurses' Association
ANS	Advances in Nursing Science
DHHS	Department of Health and Human Services
EB	*Encyclopedia of Bioethics,* ed. Warren T. Reich, NY, Free Press, 1978.
HCR	Hastings Center Report
HSA	Health Systems Agency
JNE	Journal of Nursing Education
JNM	Journal of Nurse-Midwifery
LPN	Licensed Practical Nurse
LVM	Licensed Vocational Nurse
MCN	Journal of Maternal Child Nursing
NEJM	New England Journal of Medicine
NO	Nursing Outlook
PSRO	Professional Standards Review Organization
RN	Registered Nurse
TCN	Topics in Clinical Nursing
TTB	Thompson & Thompson, *Bioethical Decision Making for Nurses*
TTE	Thompson & Thompson, *Ethics in Nursing*
WWAN	*Who's Who in American Nursing,* ed. Jeffrey Franz; Washington, D.C.: Society of Nursing Professional, 1984.

SECTION I
INTRODUCTION

CHAPTER 1

ETHICS FOR PROFESSIONAL NURSES

This text is not intended as a introduction to bioethics though the first essay gives working definitions of ethics and bioethics. The editors are principally concerned with encouraging nurses to study ethics as essential to the profession of nursing. The essay on "Nurses and the Study of Ethics" offers the pro and con views of this issue. The other chapters highlight several dimensions of it.

A part of the confusion for nurses and ethics is the concept that nurses do not need a nursing ethic because physicians already have an ethic which applies to the nursing profession. One section considers this distinction while another section looks at the decision-making process. Some people do not think nurses should make decisions and decisions have often been officially left to the physicians. Others note the day by day decisions which are made by nurses. A new sense of professional responsibility on the part of nurses has brought the nursing profession to the fore in expecting and even demanding that nurses be an official part of the decision-making process. The process itself is not always clear, however, so we include some thoughts on decision making.

Professionalism suggests that nurses are something more than employees whose only purpose is to carry out the orders or decisions of others. Not even the armed forces can claim such blatant authority anymore, so it is not surprising that today's professional nurse expects to be a part of the decision making, a part of the health care team, an equal partner in the health care professions. This has implications for relationships with physicians and change is in the wind. While traditional nursing has always cared for the patient, these changes affect that relationship also. For one thing, patient rights have taken a stronger turn and at least some patients claim a share in their own care and decisions, rather than simply following the doctor's orders, or, the nurse's orders. The relationship of nurses with nurses also stands in a new ethical light. In part this is a new understanding of the hierarchy within the nursing field, but it also means new and greater responsibility within the profession—the loyalty of nurses to nurses.

It has been said that all medical care is experimental. Medical research is thus as old as medicine itself. Can one say the same about nursing? In a sense, yes. Trial and error and what works has been a part of nursing lore and education as long as there have been nurses. New occasions however, teach new ethics. The new professionalism in nursing brings with it new demands for scientific controls, careful record-keeping and research in the usual meaning of that term. This official research is hardly new for nursing. The journal, *Nursing Research,* began in 1951. But today's nurses are more apt to be involved in research than their predecessors were. One aspect of that is in the educational side of nursing. As the educational base expands, as entry level requirements for practitioners rise, research becomes more prominent in term papers, in master's theses, doctoral dissertations, research grants for practitioners and faculty, and for all who are interested in advancing the theoretical and practical expertise of the profession.

The ethics of care and experiments on human subjects has been prominent in government and public circles. If ethics is a part of research, it must first be taught. If in fact, to be professional means to be ethical as some claim, then nurses of any kind and at all levels must have an ethical awareness—they must be sensitive to the ethical dimensions of nursing. Can this be taught or is it only caught? If it can be taught, how can it be or how should it be done? At first glance, this might be seen as only a matter for teachers. But we are all of us both teachers and students. We teach others by what we hold as important. The others may be student nurses, colleagues, patients, and even our own inner selves. What we as students—undergraduates, graduate, continuing education—expect or demand we may get. If we insist on learning about ethics, we have some greater chance of its formal inclusion in the curriculum for whatever our present level of learning. However, not all are agreed on how ethics should or can be taught. So we'll consider some options in this section.

Our concluding purpose is that students (and we are either still learning or we are "dying on the vine") will find here a beginning. It will encourage them to delve more deeply into the ethical issues around us or into the ethics of their immediate field or the ethics of patient care at all ages.

CHAPTER 2

ETHICAL DILEMMAS: CONFLICTS AMONG RIGHTS, DUTIES, AND OBLIGATIONS

Sharon Jeanne Smith and Anne J. Davis

[The authors discuss the conflicts of ethical dilemmas, legal rights, ethical rights, duties, and obligations. A section on rights versus obligations considers the patient, physician, institution, and the nurse. There is a summary of what nurses can do. Among these suggestions are to form ethics committees wherever nurses work and to participate in interdisciplinary ethics committees. The committee at the Hospital of the University of Pennsylvania has nurses as members and alternates physician/nurse as chair. The ethics committee of the School of Nursing at the University of Pennsylvania is primarily made up of nurses. As the authors note, progress is slow, but possible.]

Ethical issues in nursing practice usually are explored as if they occurred in a vacuum. Yet, approximately 78% of all nurses practice in institutions as employees. As such, many are not in decision making positions, and resolving ethical problems involves varied, sometimes conflicting, obligations.

Ethical rounds offer nurse clinicians in an institutional setting an opportunity to analyze and attempt to resolve dilemmas by exploring them with nurse ethicists. In our attempts to help nurses analyze situations during ethical rounds, we have observed that confusion frequently arises in differentiating between ethical and legal rights and between duties and obligations of patients, physicians, nurses, the institution, and others, as well as in considering the limitations that such rights, duties, and obligations impose in the delivery and receipt of health care.

Nursing, currently being practiced at a time of rapid change in social and professional values, requires that nurses consider a variety of approaches to ethical decisions.

Rule ethics predominated in nursing until the past quarter century. Certain rules, usually demanding obedience to authority, were always followed.

The utilitarian approach, making a decision according to desired end results, was often evoked, but this has significantly changed as new social values have defined new ends as desirable.

Situational ethics has come to characterize modern American society, a society steeped in pragmatism and seeking a foothold as technology sometimes outstrips our capacity to deal with the ethical problems it poses. Nurses find themselves making ethical decisions out of all three of these basic approaches, an ethical pluralism that is often unreflective.

The nursing ethics literature [often] . . focused on professional codes. More recently, it has expanded to include discussions of such particular ethical dilemmas as abortion and euthanasia and such general topics as techniques for teaching ethics, the role of the nurse as an ethical agent and patient advocate, and step-by-step models for making ethical decisions.

The treatment of ethics in the context of the nurse's role within an institution is limited, though not absent. Authors dealing with these contextual issues make the following points:

1. Nurses, as employees, work under policies established by others.(1–3)
2. Conflict arises between the professional model of nursing education and the bureaucratic model of health care institutions.(1)
3. Nurses often have responsibility but not accountability and authority.(4)
4. Nurses experience role conflict and conflict with other health care professionals, especially physicians.(4–6)
5. Nurses experience conflict between meeting a patient's needs and following institutional procedures.(2,3,6)
6. Nurses generally have either limited or no input into decisions that they are responsible for implementing.(3,5,6)

Understanding the reasons why such problems exist is a first step toward developing strategies to deal with the ethical dilemmas that they generate.

A.   ETHICAL DILEMMAS: WHAT'S THE CONFLICT

Of the numerous ethical dilemmas confronting nurses, most involve one of the following types of conflict:

1. A conflict between two ethical principles one holds.

SITUATION: A nurse works on a service where patients who have received therapeutic abortions are placed. From the viewpoint of her personal ethics, the nurse maintains that abortion is unethical. But the nurse also holds an ethical conviction, personally and in accordance with the code of nursing, that all patients ought to receive good care, regardless of their condition or personal values or characteristics.

DILEMMA: The nurse is assigned to care for a patient who has had an abortion and must decide whether to accept or refuse the assignment. The nurse believes the patient's decision to have the abortion to be unethical and yet also believes that all patients should be cared for regardless of their personal values.

2. A conflict between two possible actions in which (a) there are some, not conclusive, reasons favoring a particular course of action and (b) some, not conclusive, reasons against the same course of action.

SITUATION: A nurse works as a clinical specialist in a psychiatric emergency service where professionals may legally authorize hospitalization against an individual's will, if he is a clear and present danger to himself. The client gives some evidence of suicidal intent, but he also makes it clear that he does not wish to be hospitalized.

DILEMMA: The nurse must decide whether to hospitalize the client, thereby impinging on the client's freedom, or not hospitalize the client, who might then commit suicide.

3. A conflict between a demand for an action and the need for reflection in a situation for which the present ethical training gives insufficient precedents or preparation.

SITUATION: A nurse has just started to work in a clinic where amniocentesis is regularly done. The nurse holds that abortion is ethical when amniocentesis indicates that a birth defect is present. A couple comes to the clinic for an amniocentesis to determine the sex of the child. The couple has decided to abort the fetus if it is female, since they already have three daughters and very much want a son. The nurse has never been in this situation before and has not thought out the ramifications of this use of amniocentesis.

DILEMMA: The nurse must decide whether or not to assist with this amniocentesis, the ethical possibilities of which disturb her, particularly since she has never previously considered such a situation.

4. A conflict between two equally unsatisfactory alternatives.

SITUATION: A public health nurse is responsible for counseling a pregnant woman about whether to continue medication that will likely result in a deformed child. But if the woman stops the medication, her health and life may be in danger.

DILEMMA: The nurse must decide whether to support the woman's decision to risk the fetus by continuing the medication or to risk her life by discontinuing it.

5. A conflict between one's ethical principles and one's role obligations.

SITUATION: A hospital nurse is responsible for the surgical nursing care of a patient in a methadone maintenance program. Her duties include administering the methadone. The nurse views methadone programs as unethical because they maintain the client in a state of drug dependency. On the other hand, she is obligated by both her professional and her employee roles to provide necessary care of patients assigned.

DILEMMA: The nurse must decide whether or not to refuse the assignment to give methadone to this patient.

The employed nurse confronts such conflicts in the context of health care institutions characterized by a variety of health care professionals and legal requirements, not in a social or institutional vacuum. The nurse may use a variety of criteria for ethical decision making and then may find it is difficult and, at times, impossible to implement the ethical decision. Why does this happen?

B.   RIGHTS, DUTIES, OBLIGATIONS: WHAT'S THE DIFFERENCE?

There has been confusion in the nursing ethics literature regarding legal and ethical rights. Authors either confuse these rights or do not distinguish between them at all.

Legal Rights

Legal rights are claims recognized as valid by the legal system. Feinberg identifies four types of legal bases for claims that exist on a continuum from most to least assured and protected.(7)

1. A guaranteed legal right (a) grants legal permission for an act, (b) guarantees protection from interference by others, and (c) cannot be withdrawn even with advance notice.

EXAMPLE: A patient is brought to an emergency room after an automobile accident in which he hit his head. The physician recommends that the patient remain in the hospital for observation for 24 hours. The patient refuses to stay. The patient has a legal right to refuse further treatment.

2. A nonabsolute legal right gives both (a) permission and (b) protection for an act, but (c) is subject to interest balancing tests and thus may be withdrawn when the state finds it useful to do so.

EXAMPLE: A woman is brought to the emergency room with a bleeding ulcer. According to medical judgment, a blood transfusion is necessary or the patient will die. However, the patient refuses the transfusion on religious grounds. If the patient, who is the sole support of three minor children, dies, the children will become wards of the state. The usual right to religious liberty, invoked in the refusal of the blood transfusion, is withdrawn without prior warning because the state finds that it is in the interest of both the state and the minor children that the children continue to be cared for by the parent.

3. The legal privilege (a) grants legal permission to act, (b) may or may not provide protection from interference, but (c) both the permission to act and protection from interference, where it exists, can be withdrawn at any time (although the privilege holder will usually be warned in advance).

EXAMPLE: Shortly after a nurse gives a digitalis preparation to a patient with a pulse of 50 per minute the patient develops a cardiac arrest and dies. The case is investigated by the state board of nursing, and a hearing to consider revoking the license is called. The nursing license grants legal permission and protection to the licensee to practice nursing, but it may be withdrawn with prior warning if the nurse has vioated the conditions of licensure. The permission and protection of the license is withdrawn based on the judgment that the nurse has violated the condition of the license to practice safely.

4. A legal liberty provides (a) permission to act, but (b) no protection from interference by others.

EXAMPLE: A nurse teaches and recommends to a patient a relaxation exercise that may reduce the need for pain medication. The physician orders a pain medication to be administered at regular intervals, and the patient accepts the medicine. Unless the health teaching and counseling are specified in the nursing practice act, the nurse only has a legal liberty to teach the patient relaxation exercises. However, the physician has the legal privilege to prescribe pain medication and the patient has at least a nonabsolute legal right to accept or refuse either relaxation exercises or medication. The nurse's legal liberty to teach is not protected from interference.

Ethical Rights

An ethical right is also the basis for a claim, but the claim is called for by ethical principles or an enlightened conscience and not necessarily by legal rules. These ethical rights may or may not be upheld in a court. There are three types of ethical rights that can be viewed on a continuum from most to least widely practiced and accepted in society.

1. A conventional ethical right is a claim derived from customs, traditions, and expectations that have been established regardless of law.

EXAMPLE: In a state where privilege is not specified by law, there is an established custom that patient-nurse health care communications are confidential. The patient has an ethical right to expect the nurse will maintain confidentiality.

2. An ideal ethical right may not, in fact, be actual. It is a claim of what ought to be and what probably would be a conventional right in a "better" or ideal system.

EXAMPLE: The right to equal health care has received much recent attention. Equal access to equally excellent health care is considered an ideal ethical right of all by some members of society.

3. A conscientious ethical right is a claim that may not be recognized as valid according to either conventions or ideal rules. It is a claim based on the principles of an enlightened conscience.

EXAMPLE: In the past, some emergency rooms refused to examine patients because they were not Caucasians. These patients had a conscientious ethical right to examination. In recent years, this conscientious ethical right has become a legal right.

Duties and Obligations

Along with legal and ethical rights, one must consider legal and ethical duties and obligations.(8) Legal duties and obligations are those called for by law. Ethical duties and obligations are based on ethical principles, may or may not be called for by law, and may even be forbidden by law.

Legal duties and obligations are toward those persons and institutions defined in the law. For the nurse, these are usually patients, health care institutions, and other health professionals. Ethical duties and obligations, while not necessarily legislated, are usually toward these same groups and may be extended to include families and friends of patients and society in general.

A legal duty relates to one's role, status, or position. It is often defined in terms of rules and outlined in legislation. The nursing practice act and state board regulations define a nurse's legal duties to the patient and the state.

One incurs a legal obligation when one establishes a contract in the light of one's duties. A nurse assumes a legal obligation to fulfill the legislated duties of a registered nurse when she, as an independent practitioner, agrees to provide nursing care to a client. When a nurse is employed in a facility, that nurse assumes a legal obligation to the facility as well as to the clients assigned to her care.

One may hold certain personal ethical "principles," but an ethical "duty" is based on role, status, or position. A code of ethics delineates ethical duties for members of a profession. These ethical duties may coincide with legal duties, but they may also oblige the individual to perform more than the law requires. The *"ANA Code for Nurses"* and the *"International Code of Nursing Ethics"* define the ethical duties of nurses to clients, to the profession, and to society [Ed. Note: see Appendix]. These ethical duties are often not specified in codes of law.

One incurs an ethical obligation when one establishes a relationship based on a commitment that relates to an ethical duty. A nurse incurs an ethical obligation by virtue of the relationship formed with the patient, the institution, and other health care professionals and perhaps, the patient's family and friends and society.

Obviously, legal and ethical rights, duties, and obligations can and do conflict. That which is legal may also be considered ethical or unethical and that which is ethical may be legal or illegal. These conflicts account for a number of ethical dilemmas found in our lives both as individuals and as professional nurses. . . . (See Figure 2.1.)

	LEGAL	ILLEGAL
ETHICAL	Ethical and Legal Example: Informed Consent	Ethical and Illegal Example: Euthanasia
UNETHICAL	Unethical and Legal Example: Abortion	Unethical and Illegal Example: Involuntary Medical Treatment in a Nonemergency Situation

Figure 2.1 Conflicts between law and ethics can produce dilemmas. The problem is that which is legal may or may not be considered ethical and that which is considered ethical may or may not be legal.

C.   RIGHTS VS. OBLIGATIONS: WHO HAS WHAT?

In health care institutions, the legal and ethical rights, duties, and obligations of various parties—the patient, physician, institution, and nurse—often differ. In general, those ascribed to the nurse also apply to most other nonphysician health care professionals.

Patient

The patient has at least a nonabsolute legal right to seek health care during an illness and to accept or refuse the recommendations of health care providers. He has both a conventional and ideal ethical right to receive assistance, regardless of ability to pay.

Patients have no legal duties as health care recipients defined by legislation. The patient's only identifiable legal obligation is a civil one—to pay the bills. His primary ethical obligation is most probably to himself. However, the patient may see himself as forming an ethical contract with the physician or institution and assume an ethical duty, imposed by his own ethical principles, to cooperate in the treatment plan and follow the recommendations he has sought.

Physicians

The physician's license grants at least a legal privilege to provide medical services to patients and a legal liberty to select the setting and approach for providing services.

A conventional ethical right exists to refuse to treat in nonemergency situations if the patient refuses to follow the treatment recommendations and other health care is available. As a health care professional, the physician's primary legal and ethical duty and obligation is to the patient with whom he or she has contracted to provide service. However, the physician has the legal liberty to break the contract if the patient does not cooperate in treatment or does not reimburse the physician. And, physicians who provide medical services as employees have legal and ethical obligations to the institution.

Institution

The institution has a legal privilege and liberty and a conventional ethical right to maintain facilities for providing health care. Legal duties are present in governmental agency regulations and written contracts and agreements. Ethical duties are identified in such professional codes as the American Hospital Association's "Statement on a Patient's Bill of Rights." The institution has primary legal and ethical obligations to the patient, to its employees, and to its governing body.

Nurses

The nurse's license grants at least a legal privilege to provide services defined as nursing in the practice act. She also has a legal privilege and liberty to provide other health care services not specifically defined as nursing. However, both in and out of institutions, the protection for nurses from interference by others in the exercise of legal privilege and liberties is usually less than that accorded to physicians. Conventional ethical rights exist for some aspects of nursing care, such as confidentiality of communication, but many aspects of nursing practice rest on ideal ethical rights. As a professional health care provider, the nurse has a primary ethical obligation to the patient. However, she has legal obligations to both the institution and to the patient. Often, the nurse's implementation of professional legal and ethical duties may be hampered by the legal privilege and conventional ethical rights of the physician who is considered to have ultimate accountability for patient care or by institutional limits on the nurse's authority to act.

D.   WHAT CAN NURSES DO?

These conflicts not only exist, but they are confusing and complicated, and they form a significant source of ethical dilemmas for nurses.

Social and institutional structure and role conflict further complicate these matters. Nurses often find themselves mired in a myriad of ethical dilemmas arising from the conflict among legal and ethical rights, duties, and obligations.

What, then, can nurses do in the face of this situation? First, they should understand that laws and ethical values change slowly; the conflicts that currently exist probably will not change soon. In the past, bioethical issues and the process for ethical decision making have been discussed as if they occurred in a social and institutional vacuum. To change this, there is a need for dialogue between nurse clinicians and nurse ethicists. Such dialogue must be based on the following:

1. Education regarding legal and ethical issues to enable nurses and nursing students to better understand the dilemmas they face;

2. Integration of ethics into the curriculum of nursing schools so that ethical issues can be consistently examined and solutions sought throughout the student's clinical experiences;
3. Integration of ethics in staff development programs of health care institutions to assist nurses to examine their own ethical values and develop strategies for dealing with the ethical dilemmas they face in their practice;
4. Establishment of a standing committee on nursing ethics in the nursing services of health care institutions to assist individual nurses experiencing ethical dilemmas in understanding and attempting to resolve them.

In addition to dialogue within nursing, there is a need for interdisciplinary ethics committees within health care institutions to deal with the variety of issues and perspectives involved in today's ethical dilemmas. Members of a nursing ethics committee should sit on the interdisciplinary committees to provide a means of communication between nursing personnel and other disciplines and levels of the institutional hierarchy.(9)

ENDNOTES

1. Margaret O'Brien Steinfels, "Ethics, Education, and Nursing Practice," HCR 7 (Aug 77), 20–21.

2. Catherine P. Murphy, "The Moral Situation in Nursing," pp. 313–320 in Bioethics and Human Rights ed. Elsie L. and Bertram Bandman; Boston: Little, Brown, 1978.

3. Bandman and Bandman, "Do Nurses Have Rights?," AJN 78 (Jan 78), 84–86.

4. Andrew Jameton, "The Nurse: When Roles and Rules Conflict," HCR 7 (Aug 77), 22–23.

5. K. Boyd, "The Nature of Ethics," Nursing Mirror 145 (21 July 77), 14–16.

6. M. Bunzl, "A Note on Nursing Ethics in the USA," Journal of Medical Ethics 1 (Dec 75), 184–186.

7. Joel Feinberg, "Rights," pp. 38–43 in Contemporary Issues in Bioethics ed. Tom L. Beauchamp and LeRoy Walters; Belmont, CA: Dickenson, 1978.

8. John Lemmon, "Moral Dilemmas," pp. 6–11, Beauchamp and Walters, op. cit. [ed.: Neither Feinberg, n. 7, nor Lemmon, are included in Beauchamp and Walters, 2nd ed.; Belmont: Wadsworth, 1982.]

9. The authors wish to thank the nurses of the University of California Hospital, San Francisco, wards 5A and B, who, while participating in nursing ethics rounds, raised the concerns that led to this paper.

SECTION II
NURSES AND THE STUDY OF ETHICS

CHAPTER 3

WHY SHOULD NURSES STUDY ETHICS?

Joyce E. Thompson and Henry O. Thompson

["No" is one answer to the question of whether nurses should study ethics, and there are a number of reasons for this answer. The authors, on the other hand, answer "Yes" and discuss the outcome. Nurses work with people, make decisions, serve in health care teams that make decisions, and have professional status. There are implications for individual nurses as well as the profession of nursing.]

AN HISTORICAL PERSPECTIVE

There are many people outside the profession of nursing, and others within who would answer the question, "Should nurses study ethics?" with an emphatic, "No!" When reasons are given, they often vary on the theme that nurses do not make decisions. The almost complete lack of references to nurses in medical ethics literature could be interpreted to support this negative view.

Nurses Do Not Make Decisions

One could trace the origin of this reasoning to the history of nursing and to the feminine role in nursing the sick. Florence Nightingale clearly defined the role of the nurse as "servant"—to the physician, to the client, to others. Nurses in the past and many today accept the "handmaiden" role. Following orders without question has been the rule more often than not.

Nursing has often been thought of as a female profession. Women have been socialized to be dependent, subservient, the passive member in the female-male relationship. This has carried over to the health care

Reprinted from *Scholar & Educator,* Spring 1984, 8, no. 1, 51–61. Used with permission of authors.

system where most physicians are men and most nurses are women.(1) It has been comfortable—socially acceptable—for nurses to follow the doctor's orders. In addition, it has meant they did not have to make the effort to decide and did not have to take responsibility for decisions. The feminist movement of today has brought or is beginning to bring changes in these traditional roles. Nurses are taking responsibility for decisions. There is an increasing respect for nurses as persons.

Nurse-Physician Relationship

Until recently, the legal system has supported the traditional system. Physicians were held accountable under the law. Colloquially, the "buck stopped with the physician" rather than the nurse. The health care system has also contributed to the traditional pattern. Clients contract with the physician rather than the nurse. Nurses "come along with the package" of hospital or health care. Both systems suggest the physician is ultimately responsible and nurses are told repeatedly they must defer to "doctor's orders." Nurses have been fired for "interfering with the patient-physician relationship." Perhaps more commonly they have been given less pleasant work assignments, transferred to unacceptable duty shifts or harassed in other ways. Individual nurses who were concerned with the patient's welfare rather than the physician's best interests found little or no support from the *nursing* hierarchy. The result has been a predictable passivity with the aphorism that "you can't fight the system."

Covert Decisions

The system has not, however, stopped nurses from making decisions. These are rather made without open admission. Sometimes nurses themselves do not realize what they are doing. For example, nurses learn which physician will support what the nurse wants or thinks is best for patient care. If they are turned down by one, they may proceed to another. Some of these "games" are power struggles. Nurses may think they know best what a client needs, and may be right. However, if such covert decisions are only for power, the patient may end up with the battle scars.

Another example of covert decisions is speed of response. One nurse may not want to be involved in a decision about resuscitation but thinks it should be done. That nurse moves quickly when a patient arrests. Another may think it should not be done and move slowly. One of the ethical problems with this and all covert decisions is lack of responsibility for the decisions. It also involves a failure to move the system to more ethical decision making. It may prevent further learning about ethical decision making. It may also, however, mean more ethical care for patients when the system is lax or simply fails.

Priority for Study

A different kind of decision may take place in nursing education on the study of ethics. How much can be done in an already overcrowded curriculum? The knowledge explosion means setting priorities. Of course, the choices reflect the moral beliefs and the ethical standards of the persons involved and the nursing profession as a whole. Very few nursing education programs require the study of ethics although a large number allow it. The lack of requirement suggests a negative answer to the question, "should nurses study ethics?"

Motivational Factors

A final point is the simple reality that a nurse may not wish to study ethics. The study may be difficult and complex. Some ethical dilemmas do not have easy answers. Ethics itself has a complex variety of theological, philosophical, and technological concepts. Nurses, like many people, tend to function in concrete ways rather than abstract ones. Health care may be a matter of diet, or type of dressing, rather than a philosophical ideal. Ethics do not always, and some would say rarely, deal with absolutes. An ethical dilemma may require a choice between two or more actions that appear equally right or wrong. This can be frustrating. Some nurses are content or comfortable following orders or implementing the decisions of others. They may be "appliance" nurses—working long enough to earn the money for a new household appliance. Motivation for work can determine willingness to study ethics. An ethical decision has already been made if the job has been given priority, whether for an appliance or if an individual *must* work for a living. There is no conflict for the nurse between patients' rights and employer's rights for the decision has already been made. One may not see any reason for studying the pro or con of a decision which has already been made.

AN AFFIRMATIVE RESPONSE

Our position is that nurses should study ethics. Nurse work with people. Nurses make decisions every day, perhaps every hour, that affect the health and the very life of people. Nurses should be responsible members of the health care team. Nursing is or ought to be a profession and nurses should be practicing in a professional manner. It has been said that to be professional is to be ethical and vice versa.(2) Each of these attributes support the study of ethics.

Working with People

One of the central goals of nursing is to care for people with respect and dignity, supporting the client's right to self-determination.(3) Nurses have a covenant relationship with their patients. Nurses are not to abandon a patient regardless of the health problem involved. This covenant may not be easy to maintain when the client and nurse disagree on some issue such as the use of resources, euthanasia, abortion, etc. Clients bring with them a variety of beliefs, values, customs, and moral positions along with their health needs. And of course, nurses do also. The nurse's professional responsibilities for practice are factored into this multifaceted relationship. Kelly(4) notes that people who choose nursing as a career make a commitment to their clients that goes beyond their own personal feelings and moral standards. This professional commitment is included in the ANA *Code for Nurses with Interpretive Statements.*(5) In order to respect the patient, nurses need to know what these beliefs, etc., are, and how these might influence the client's ability to request, receive or refuse health care.(6)

Nurses also need to understand their own value system. This can influence the nurse-patient relationship and the manner in which professional nursing is provided. Understanding the nature of values, including one's own, is central to the study of ethics.(7) One reason for nurses to study ethics is to begin to identify their own moral positions and biases. Then they need to explore ways to prevent these biases from unconsciously interfering with the ability to provide care. Values clarification is important for nurses making ethical decisions. It is not the same as making ethical decisions. Nurses who know and understand what they believe and value will not necessarily make ethical decisions. Circumstances may require or promote actions inconsistent with the nurse's own values. The nurse's values may be inconsistent with those of others: patients, physicians, other nurses, etc.

Nurses Make Decisions

These decisions may or may not be the headline catchers, such as not to give treatment to a defective neonate. They are decisions affecting other people. The need for nurses in the headline cases is crucial and will be discussed later. Here we note that there are many decisions by nurses. As nurses continue to expand their practice to primary care, even more decisions will be required.(8) Today's nurse can maintain an ethical perspective by being aware that all decisions have an ethical dimension. Nurses are working with people and nurses make decisions affecting others and themselves as well.

There are many questions that commonly occur. What ought to be done in this situation? Is this action in the best interest of the client? Who should make the decision? Who decides who decides? What is the right thing to do? What harm or benefit will come from the decision and the resulting actions? If we can, should we? Does the nurse have a right to disagree with the client's or physician's decision? What rights does the institution or society have if we follow a specific action? Should negligent actions be reported if no harm has resulted?

Ethical dilemmas may arise when client and professional values differ.(9) These dilemmas require a responsible choice between two or more actions, often of equal rightness or wrongness, as defined by the people involved. Such choices need a clear understanding of the values that motivate behavior, their sources, and implications.(10) Other questions that indicate a value conflict also come up. If a nurse is not comfortable about a decision made by a colleague or client, what steps if any should s/he take? Does a nurse have a right to take further action? On what grounds? Does a "scientific" treatment take precedence over a holistic or natural approach?(11) If a patient has not been told the truth by the physician, should the nurse tell her? How a nurse responds reflects the nurse's own moral standard. That includes setting priorities in decision making. Such priority setting is also an ethical decision. The study of ethics can help nurses understand what is involved. In turn, this can lead to ethical and knowledgeable participation in decision making.

Medical ethics literature rarely mentions the nurse in the stellar, headline cases. The nurse's relationship with the patient involves the most continuous contact time. Thus nurses may have vital knowledge about the patient and the family that should be considered when deciding a course of action. It is often the nurses who carry out the decision made by the team. Without input and understanding why the decision was made, the nurse may be confused or ineffectual. That is doubly so when a nurse disagrees with a decision. There is also an ethical question of simple justice or fairness. A decision is made for no further treatment, without nursing consultation. The physician leaves and requests no further discussion. The family goes home to grieve and get on with their lives. The nurse is left to stand by and watch the end. Fairness suggests that the people who make the decision should have the responsibility of carrying it out.

Team Membership

Nurses have a variety of roles during their career. These roles may be alone or in combination with others. They may include advocate, counselor, confidant, caregiver, decision-maker, colleague, or team leader. The nature of nursing requires concern for patients and their families, colleagues in health care, the institution or employer, society as a whole, and one's self. These roles have ethical components within which actions might be taken.(12) They can also result in conflicts. The competent professional is concerned with them all, while recognizing that at a given moment, there may be priorities. These priorities and ethical components are yet another reason for nurses to study ethics.

With the expansion of nursing practice into primary care, more nurses are recognizing and taking responsibility for making health care decisions, usually in collaboration with the patient/family. While the law changes more slowly, individual nurses have welcomed the direct responsibility. State licensing laws for nurse practitioners are often written in terms of physician supervision implying physician responsibility. The reality is that physicians are not always present, nor do they need to be. Nurses are in direct contact with clients and are competently making many of the decisions.

Team Decisions

Some have suggested that the way to ensure ethical decisions and the best interests of the patient is to have these decisions made through team discussion and action.(13) These are often the stellar decisions on life and death where there may be time to have a meeting and discussion. Reviews "after the fact" of decisions made in an emergency can be a learning opportunity for the team. Members of the group may face similar decisions in the future. Even though reviews may not help the situation which has past, they may help people live with that past; that includes distinguishing the uniqueness of the situation as well as commonalities with other situations.

The team for decision making or review may include the client, family, clergy, nurse, doctor, social worker, others. Mutual respect is required for the team to function. So is a level of trust conducive to sharing feelings and value systems. The emphasis here is on understanding colleagues' values as well as those of the client and family. This of course takes time and effort but, in turn, can develop the level of respect needed and result in more ethical decisions.

Professional Status

The idea of a profession has many angles, such as being ethical as cited earlier. For discussion purposes, we note here the two concepts of accountability for actions and for maintaining competence in nursing practice as elements of the nursing profession's ethics. The latter includes updating knowledge and the expansion of skills as well as simply maintaining them. The ANA *Code for Nurses* is a resource for defining the ethical scope of such competence. Some do not think nursing has attained the status of a profession. Others think the professional status began with Florence Nightingale. The issues of accountability and competence are important for both.

Many nurses today accept accountability. As responsible professionals, they learn about the legal and ethical implications of their practice. There are still institutions, employers, colleagues and some clients who interfere with some nurses' willingness to make decisions responsibly. At times, these same persons are quick to hold nurses responsible when something goes wrong or goes against the establishment. Some nurses are willing to take a stand for their actions instead of acquiescing to institutional or colleague priorities to the detriment of patient care. To blindly follow orders without regard to patient welfare does not reflect responsible, accountable nursing practice. To openly decide and to admit that one took an action because "in my best judgment" it was what the patient needed, is to be accountable. "In my best judgment" is, of course, a value loaded statement. Whether the judgment was ethical depends on many factors such as clear and accurate identification of patient needs, informed consent, and the ethical theory used to rule on the ethicalness of the decision.

The need to maintain competency is almost taken for granted. This is not always true, however, for bioethics. This is itself a rapidly expanding field requiring decisions which has led to the development of new technologies for keeping people alive, producing healthier babies, enhancing the quality of life, etc. One question that comes up concerns the "is—ought" issue. Because we can keep someone alive, should we? Another asks about the cost to the family or to society? While some issues are newer than this morning's headlines, others are as old as the dawn of time, tempered only by the societal values of today and those of the individuals involved. Questions of theft or murder, what is the loving thing to do, how to do good and to avoid harm, are issues that have been around for a long time but now have new dimensions.

Nurses who work in critical care or research units may be more familiar with the kind of dilemmas raised by technology. When should a patient be put on a respirator may be as difficult an issue as when should such equipment be withdrawn? Whether amniocentesis should be required of all women is more complex than a simple yes or no answer. A few decades ago, such decisions were less common. The technology was not available to offer such options. With their more constant contact with patients, nurses have been closely affected by the dilemmas of technology. Responsible decision making requires knowledge. The study of ethics is one way to gain the knowledge needed for ethical decisions.

IMPLICATIONS FOR THE INDIVIDUAL NURSE

When nurses choose to study ethics, including values clarification and ethical theories, many things can happen. One of the most exciting, yet potentially threatening, is that individuals will begin to know themselves, perhaps even more than one wishes. This self-revelation is exciting for those interested in continued growth as an individual as well as a nurse. One important aspect of values clarification for nurses is caring for people with opposing values or morals. Caring for drug addicts, suicidal people, prostitutes, or people electing plastic surgery to alter body appearance may be difficult for a nurse who cannot accept their choices. Both nurse and client will benefit when the nurse knows what will be tolerated so that good care results, and from which situations the nurse must withdraw, making sure a colleague assumes care responsibilities so that poor care does not result. The *Code for Nurses* implies that the individual nurse should work well with all patients (Statement 1). This may not always be possible.

Another potential outcome of the study of ethics for nurses is awareness of the difficulty of "walking in the shoes of the physician" where the "buck stops." Nurses have had the opportunity to "pass the buck" of difficult decisions to the physician. The physician does not usually have that option. One result of realizing the difficulty of making ethical decisions is greater respect for others. Mature, collegial relationships are possible when all team members see one another as people with a variety of beliefs and values, working together for the common good in an ethical manner.

Of course, the opposite side of the decision-making experience is that nurses who once demanded more input and autonomy may wish they had not been heard. Making difficult decisions does not always win friends, and sometimes those decisions are wrong in retrospect. A sense of maturity is required for all involved, including a willingness for critical reflection on past actions as well as team discussion of future ones.

IMPLICATIONS FOR THE PROFESSION OF NURSING

As nurses study ethics and participate more actively in ethical decisions, the profession will gain greater respect among other professions and with clients. The study of ethics is implicit in nursing education that focuses on accountability and the expansion of practice into primary care activities. The new image of the professional nurse is one who has competence and autonomy and who develops mature collegial relationships while working toward the goal of quality health and illness care for all people. The study of ethics can help nurses achieve this new image by preparing them for practice in an ethical manner through self-awareness, through a willingness to make decisions openly and by accepting responsibility.

The concept, "to be professional is to be ethical or to be ethical is to be professional," is deeper than external respect. Without ethics there is no profession of nursing. If nursing expects to have a future as a profession, then it must be ethical. Nurses must know ethics, the ethical perspective, what it means to be ethical. Without that knowledge, nursing has no future as a profession; it can only continue the "handmaiden" image of the past.

SUMMARY

In conclusion, we do not choose to summarize the above discussion so much as to lift up a new vision of collegiality hinted at in these pages. For those who have known a type of pseudo-authority over others, this new collegiality may be threatening. As nurses request, yea claim, accountability as professionals, others may fear this as an invasion of territory—their turf. There is an alternative perspective that touches upon the woman/man relationship mentioned earlier which includes the whole concept of authority. It is not only more ethical, but more enriching and exciting for people to work together as equals with due respect for each other's expertise, rather than in a servant and master relationship. This is, of course, a value statement.

ENDNOTES

1. Malcah T. Nottman & Carol C. Natelson, "Women as Patients and Experimental Subjects," EB IV:1704–1713. Natelson & Nottman, "Women as Health Professionals," EB IV:1713–1720.

2. Personal communication, Donald Jones, Drew University, Madison, NJ.

3. *Code for Nurses with Interpretive Statement;* Kansas City, MO: ANA, 1986.

4. Lucie Kelly, *Dimensions of Professional Nursing,* 3rd ed.; NY: Macmillan, 1975, pp. 208–220.

5. ANA, op. cit.

6. R.C. Dilday, "The Code for Nurses: An Educational Perspective," pp. 10–17 in *ANA Perspective on the Code for Nurses;* Kansas City, MO: ANA, 1978.

7. Shirley Steele & Vera Harmon, *Values Clarification in Nursing,* 2nd ed; Norwalk, CT: Appleton-Century-Crofts, 1983. Anne Davis & Mila A. Aroskar, *Ethical Dilemmas and Nursing Practice,* 2nd ed.; Norwalk, CT: Appelton-Century-Crofts, 1983.

8. Paula Sigman, "Ethical Choices in Nursing," ANS 1, No. 2 (Ap 79), 37–52. Lucie Kelly, "Endpaper: Can't Can't," NO 27, No. 7 (July 79), 496.

9. Rita Payton, "Nurse-practitioners and Ethics in Practice," presentation, National Conference for Nurse-Practitioners; Keystone, CO: June 79.

10. Claire Jacobi, "Dilemmas for Educators: Values or Valuing," *Kappa Delta Pi Record* 12, No. 2 (Dec 75), 50–51. Sigman, op. cit., p. 42.

11. Norman Cousins, "The Doctor-Patient Relationship," *Man & Medicine* 4, No. 2 (1979), 121–127. Sr. A. Teresa Stanley, "Is it Ethical to Give Hope to a Dying Person?," *Nursing Clinics of North America* 14, No. 1 (May 79), 69–80.

12. Andrew Jameton, "The Nurse: When Roles and Rules Conflict," HCR 7, No. 4 (Aug 77), 22–23. "Nursing Ethics: The Admirable Professional Standards of Nurses—A Survey Report," *Nursing* 74, No. 9 (Sep 74), 35.

13. Sylvia Gendrop, "The Order: No Code," *Linacre Quarterly* 44, No. 4 (Nov 77), 313. Dagmar Cechanek, "Nursing Reactions," pp. 59–60 in *Ethical Dilemmas in Current Obstetric and Newborn Care,* Report of the 65th Ross Conference on Pediatric Research, ed. Tom D. Moore; Columbus, OH: 1973. Norman Fost & John Robertson, "Letter to the Editor," NEJM 295, No. 20 (1976), p. 1141.

CHAPTER 4

THE NURSE AS ADVOCATE: A PHILOSOPHICAL FOUNDATION FOR NURSING

Leah L. Curtin

[Nursing is moving toward the medical model with its emphasis on science and technology and moving out of nursing with its emphasis on human beings. Curtin offers an alternative to this hi tech philosophy. Nursing is a moral art concerned with human decency. Disease damages our humanity with loss of freedom and choice. Nurses as patient advocates are concerned with the restoration of humanness, not only in serious matters but in daily living. The nurse-patient relationship is the essence of nursing.]

Nurses seem to be moving in the direction of the medical model with its emphasis on science, technology and cure. As individual nurses and as members of a profession we are seeking fundamental clarifications and asking radical questions. In partial reaction to this move toward the medical we seem to be diverting to what is essentially a historical model of nursing with an emphasis on an intuitive approach. The answers that we reach, the direction that we choose will determine the future parameters of nursing.

Some sociologists have suggested that rather than developing as nursing professionals, professional nurses are evolving out of nursing! "Nursing will still be nursing, but it will be carried on by persons of other occupational affiliations."(1) What then will nurses be doing while someone else is doing nursing?

According to some nursing leaders, nurses will be moving on to "meta-nursing." Travelbee claims that "The role of the nurse must be transcended in order to relate as human being to human being."(2) If

Reprinted from *Advances in Nursing Science*, vol. 1, no. 3, pp. 1–10, with permission of Aspen Publishers, Inc., copyright April 1979.

the role of the nurse is viewed in such a manner, it is no wonder that nurses wish to move on to better things.

What is nursing? What is the role of the nurse? What is it that makes a nurse a nurse? Is it indeed the functions that we perform? How is it then that the director of nursing service, the administrator of a nursing home, the dean of a college of nursing, the primary care nurse, the operating room nurse, the public health nurse, the psychiatric nurse all claim to be nurses? We perform radically different functions and yet each of us claims the title "nurse." How can it be that those who, in the eyes of sociologists, have moved beyond nursing still consider themselves nurses? Could it be that rather than evolving out of nursing, these nurses are actualizing new possibilities within nursing?

Could it be that nursing *should not* be defined sociologically, but rather philosophically? Nursing can and should be distinguished by its philosophy of care and *not* by its care functions. Nurses themselves must formulate this philosophy and when they do, they transcend any particular function of nursing only to realize a more developed concept—a concept that embraces and unifies the experience of all nurses rather than denying or denigrating any of that experience.(3)

A.   NURSING—A MORAL ART

The end or purpose of nursing is the welfare of other human beings. This end is not a scientific end, but rather a moral end. That is, it involves the seeking of good and it involves our relationship with other human beings. The science that we learn, the technological skills that we develop are both shaped and designed by that moral end—much as an artist uses a brush. Therefore, nursing is a moral art.(4) The wise and human application of our knowledge and skill is the moral art of nursing. Nursing science serves this art, and this art would not be possible without nursing science. This art is a moral art because it involves other human beings, our relationship with those human beings and the promotion of what we see mutually as "good"—health.

The Concept of Advocacy

Anyone acquainted with the history of nursing is familiar with the various models proposed as models of nursing, such as the nurse as caretaker, the nurse as champion of the sick, the nurse as health educator, the nurse as physician assistant (extender, surrogate, etc.), the nurse as parent surrogate, and the nurse as healer. None of these seems adequate.

Perhaps the philosophical foundation and ideal of nursing is the nurse as advocate. The concept of advocacy implied here is not the concept implied in the patients' rights movement nor the legal concept of advocacy, but a far more fundamental advocacy founded upon the simplest and most basic of premises. This concept is not simply one more alternative to be added to the list of past and present concepts of nursing nor does it reject any of them—it embraces all of them. It is not structured rigidly so as to preclude alternatives, rather it involves the basic nature and purpose of the nurse-patient relationship. It is proposed as a very simple foundation upon which the nurse and patient in any given encounter can freely determine the form that relationship is to have, i.e., child and parent, client and counselor, friend and friend, colleague and colleague and so forth through the range of possibilities. This foundation is philosophically prior to any particular relationship and, in fact, enables that relationship to exist.

This proposed ideal of advocacy is based upon our common humanity, our common needs and our common human rights. We are human beings, our patients or clients are human beings, and it is this commonality that should form the basis of the relationship between us. It often seems that we have permitted traditionalism, elitism and more recently legalism to obscure this most basic of facts.

What It Means to Be a Human Being

To even begin to understand what the human relationship in the professional context means, we have to examine who we are and where we come from. We must approach these questions in the only way we know how, as individuals whose knowing begins with our senses. What we are examining are human beings, very special kinds of beings who exist in a visible ambience at a determinable point in time and space, beings who know and who know that they know, beings who laugh and cry—and sometimes know why.

Human beings cannot be fragmented. One of our deepest convictions, confirmed by all of our experience, is that each person is a unity.(5) I who think, I who know, I who feel, I who hope, I who fear, I who believe am one! As we grow and mature we come to realize that although we are separate and distinct from all other creatures in the world, we belong to them and with them because we have grown out of the growth of others, learned from their knowledge and benefited from their sufferings. Each person is an integrity, a unity, but a unity that is interrelated and interdependent.

Slowly and painfully, we have come to understand and demand our own dignity. We now know that freedom, respect and integrity are essential to our full development as persons. These concepts have crystallized in what we call human rights.(6) Although it has taken us a bit longer, we now realize that these rights belong to all persons—young and old, black, white, red and yellow; healthy and sick. The progress in this direction has not been smooth, nor is there anything to keep us from backsliding, but progress has been made.(7)

These concepts we call human rights derive essentially from human needs—*not* human wants, but real, fundamental human needs. Whether the right is physical (such as the right to bodily integrity) or intellectual (such as the right to learn), each is essential to our integrity—or our unity—as persons.

B. HUMAN RIGHTS AND THE NURSE-PATIENT RELATIONSHIP

The relevance of this concept of human rights to the nurse-patient relationship is profound because the patient/client's human needs are magnified by disease. Moreover, the process of the disease itself renders the patient/client far more vulnerable to abuse. Furthermore, the disease process itself may well create new, fundamental needs, needs that must be addressed if the person is to maintain unity-integrity as a unique human being.

Nurses are in a unique position among health professionals to attend the patient/client as a unity because they are able to experience patients as human beings.(8) Not only do nurses attend patients when distress is immediate, but they attend them for sustained periods of time, often providing those intimate details of physical and emotional care that lead to a knowledge of this person as a distinct and unique human being. This knowledge is a precondition for the fundamental type of advocacy referred to here— not legal advocacy, not even health advocacy, but human advocacy.

The only way in which the *unique* human needs of patients or clients can be met is for nurses to attend them as unities. This requires not only an understanding of patients as human beings, but an understanding of each patient as a unique human being. Nurses must be sensitive to individuals and to their reactions to those needs created by illness that threaten the unity or integrity of the person.

Not only must nurses understand the specific physiological damage caused by disease processes, but they must also understand what illness does to the humanity of the sufferer. The wounds produced by illness stretch far beyond the person's physiological or even psychological limits and penetrate the existential depths of the person's being.(9) These very special wounds create very special needs—needs that must be met if we are to minister to the patient as a human being. These wounds must be addressed if we are to respect the human rights of patients/clients, if we are to accept human advocacy as the foundation of the nurse-patient relationship.

C.   HOW DISEASE DAMAGES OUR HUMANITY

Loss of Independence

One of the first things that illness does to human beings is to infringe upon their autonomy or independence as people. At the very least, individuals are required to go to another person, to place themselves before this person, to admit that they have a deficiency or a defect and to ask to have it alleviated. In effect, disease makes a petitioner out of an independent individual and threatens the person's self-image. The more personal or more threatening the disclosure is, the more difficult it is for a person to reveal the problem.

Ordinarily, when we meet with a threat we either fight or flee.(10) Yet we cannot flee from ourselves, nor can we fight that within ourselves which we cannot control. This is the ultimate threat, the threat that comes from within, and no matter how hard we try, we cannot have it alleviated without becoming a petitioner. The position of a petitioner is so repugnant to many that they will go to great lengths and take great risks to avoid it. If we are sensitive to this difficulty, the pain it imposes, the humiliation it brings, we can take some steps to alleviate it. So often it seems that health professionals (and nurses are no exception) are so caught up in their own business, their own knowledge and their own self-importance that they fail to consider this first humiliation of the patient or client. We must be willing to unravel the "medical mystique," to become more accessible and to remember that we too are human beings. It is only in doing so that we can begin to heal this first wound to the humanity, to assist individuals to overcome this first obstacle.

Loss of Freedom of Action

The second wound that impinges upon the humanity of the individual is the loss of freedom of action. The human being uses the body to transcend the body itself.(11) That is, unlike animal, we use our bodies for more than the fulfillment of physiological needs and instinctual drives. Human beings are bodily creatures, but they use their bodies to express their hopes, dreams, ideals and values. When we are ill we cannot command our bodies to do what we want them to do and thus in this sense our humanity is wounded, sometimes very seriously.

Insofar as possible we must assist the patient/client to communicate these essential aspects of their humanity. If they cannot do so, we must take steps to discover their value systems and then to respect them. The losses of freedom to action (verbal, locomotive, often intellectual) inflict another wound to the individual's humanity—and sometimes a very serious one!

Interference with Ability to Make Choices

In a third dimension our humanity is damaged by the interference of disease with our ability to make choices—not our right to make choices, but our ability to exercise that right. While there are many factors operant in decision making, it still remains that a decision to be truly valid, must be rational. This is a particularly sensitive area. Often professionals may consider only those decisions that agree with their own to be rational. This is not necessarily the case. However, we must be aware that pain, disability, trauma and drugs all becloud the ability to make choices as does the trauma caused by the loss of wholeness and the loss of ability to act.

Nevertheless, in all circumstances the right to consent rests within the individual. Under certain circumstances we may presume consent; in others we may obtain authorization to act; but the right always remains within the individual. If we are sensitive to this fact, we are far more likely to try to discover and act upon the patient's value system rather than our own or that of significant others. Because this situation has been greatly magnified by our increasing technological power to intervene in an individual's life, the responsibility to discover and respect the patient's value system has assumed vastly increased significance.(12)

Power of Health Care Professionals

A corollary of these factors, and perhaps one of the most devastating attacks on our personhood, is that we are placed in the power of others. Many institutions in society exercise enormous power over us, but these powers have been recognized and surrounded with legal safeguards. It has been widely recognized, for example, that consent obtained under duress is not legally binding.(13) Few things in life are as coercive as the threat of suffering and death (in this instance imposed by illness). Yet what legal advocate, what laws of state, can protect us from these? Thus those persons whom we see as capable of relieving these threats can and do exercise enormous power over us. Not only do patients, generally speaking, lack the knowledge necessary to define the threat, but they also lack the ability to reduce the threat. Whether we as health professionals want it or not, whether we like it or not, we exercise enormous power over those whom we should serve. How do we use this power? What does this power mean in the light of human advocacy?

D. RESPONSIBILITIES OF HUMAN ADVOCACY

Information must be provided—at least enough to enable patients/ clients to choose among options; but how and when patients/clients are told are at least as significant as what they are told. In the past (and often today), patients were uninformed largely because it was assumed that the health professionals, perhaps in concert with families, knew what was best for the patients. Usually professionals do know what is best from the technical viewpoint, but it is doubtful that such knowledge extends into the realm of values.

Today, largely because of legal requirements, patients may be subjected to a tyranny of information. More as a hedge against malpractice than out of respect for human rights, patients are fed an enormous, disagreeable and indigestble lump of information—and all at one sitting. How much more patients would benefit from small amounts of information provided when they are ready for them and as they ask for them. If nurses and physicians worked collaboratively rather than jealously protecting territorial limits, the patient would greatly benefit. Because nurses have the opportunity to experience the patient as a unique human being and because they spend more time with the patient, nurses can more readily provide information as the patient requests it and when the patient is prepared for it.

Because individuals have been damaged by trauma or disease, and perhaps because they have been placed in the power of others, they have to a large extent *lost their freedom to define for themselves their own image of what it is they should be.* For example, there was a case of a 22-year-old male patient who was diagnosed as having primary cancer of the testes. He was a jockey, a husband and the father of two young sons.

There was no evidence of metastasis. He was told of his diagnosis, the need for an orchiectomy and the effect this operation would have on his relationship with his wife. He and his wife discussed the situation and, considering the alternative, decided upon surgery. What he was not told, however, was at least as significant as what he was told. He was not told that he would lose his facial hair, develop breasts and develop a feminine speaking voice. How much did we impinge upon this person's identity? What did we do to his self-image? What image did he present to his sons? To his wife? What kind of comments did he have to endure at the race track? We do not know, but what we do know is that he committed suicide nine months after surgery.

So often by trying to do what we think is right by our value system, we trespass upon the authenticity of the person. Although in many cases our transgressions are not so great, in some cases they are profound. This man's decision might not have been any different if he had known all the facts, but the real question is whether or not the *individual rather than the professional* should make such value decisions. If we decide that a person cannot, how do we reach this conclusion? Can we not, should we not, ought we not assist the patient in decision making AND YET RESPECT THE PATIENT'S DECISION once it is made?

If these wounds are not addressed, and indeed if they are exacerbated, the most devastating of existential wounds develops. Insofar as patients' values are ignored, or replaced with others' values, patients cease to exist as unique human beings. Depersonalization may be partial or complete, but those individuals will die as the persons they were. If the depersonalization is complete, those individuals will not be able to create new values and goals in their life and they will lose a sense of meaning or purpose in their existence.(14) As the philosopher Nietzsche put it, "He who has the why to live can bear with almost any how."(15)

We must—as human advocates—assist patients to find meaning or purpose in their living or in their dying. This can mean whatever the patients want it to mean; it can range from enlisting religious aid to cracking irreverent jokes, from finding a new vocation to adjusting to the old one, from fighting the inevitable to the last breath to complete acceptance of death. Whatever patients define as their goal, it is their meaning and not ours, their values and not ours, and their living or dying, not ours.

Any application of human advocacy is subject to personal and situational interpretation by the practitioner. This is precisely why human advocacy can serve as a foundation upon which any practitioner in any given situation can develop the framework of the nurse-patient relationship according to the unique needs presented by that particular relationship.

According to Garver, violence is not so much a matter of force as it is a matter of violating persons physically, intellectually or psychologically.(15) Certainly not every limitation of a person's autonomy can be seen as an act of violence. To take this position would be to take the moral "punch" out of the notion of psychological violence. For example, one simply cannot equate a regulation limiting how loud parties may tune their television sets with the rendering of patients incompetent in various degrees by withholding information, thus interfering with their rational processes. The concept of psychological violence must be reserved to those cases in which grave or systematic harm is done to the person. The ability to distinguish those cases requires a sensitivity to the human needs created by illness and the unique manifestation of these needs in each patient, NOT IN SERIOUS MATTERS ONLY, but in the daily living experience of patients/clients.

Consider the daily living experience of an institutionalized patient. An individual comes into the patient's room to insert an I.V., and the patient does not even know about the I.V. or why it is being given. Another person comes in to administer a medication that the patient does not even know about or why it is being given. Still another person comes in to catheterize the patient, to administer an enema, to draw blood, to examine every part of the patient's body, to transport the patient here or there for this test or that, and the patient doesn't even know where they are going, what is being done or why it is is being done.

Each individual violation may or may not amount to a serious infringement on the patient's autonomy, but collectively they constitute both physical and psychological violence. Note that the effect on the patient is systematic. Confusion, lack of knowledge, lack of explanation, the pervasive assumption that the patient's body belongs to the "professionals" to do with what they will—all lead to reduced possibilities for decision making. Such systematic violation leads to reduced possibilities for making decisions in other, perhaps critical, areas. Human beings are reduced to objects acted upon, in effect a whosesale reduction of autonomous decision making.(16) Patient and family are thus rapidly socialized into obedience patterns and nonconformity is swiftly punished in both subtle and not so subtle ways.

E.   ESSENCE OF NURSING

Nurses can and do control the environment of the institution, and nurses can institute progressive and humanizing changes if they so desire. Explanations and working together with a patient are not extras that nurses may choose to do, they are the essence of nursing, the essence of the nurse-patient relationship. Obviously, in certain critical situations, there is no time for an in-depth discussion of values or even explanations. These circumstances, however, constitute only a minute portion of nurse-patient interactions and should not be used to negate patient rights in the majority of situations.

To claim that nurses can institute progressive change is not to ignore the many organizational and social barriers that nurses face. We can control our own actions. To be sure there are inflexible policies and insensitive orders from physicians, but the professional nurse has a great deal of latitude in the implementation of such policies and orders. Our ethical responsibility is not reduced by the actions of others, but in fact may be magnified by them.(17) Discretion and maturity are necessary components of the truly effective professional.

Nursing and the individual nurse are in very vital positions to help create a climate respectful of the human rights and needs of patients. No other profession and no other professional can exercise as great an influence over the environment of the institution (the environment of the patient) as do the nurse and nursing. If we, as a profession, work together to create an atmosphere that is open to and supportive of the individual's decision making, we may well perform our greatest service to patients/clients and their families.

In many instances nurses are not free to disclose certain information to patients/clients and their families. That is, they are not free unless they are willing to pay the price, a price that may well include loss of employment or even licensure. This situation is wrong because it violates both the patient's and the nurse's integrity.(18) Moreover, it constitutes infringement of the nurse's right to practice nursing and interferes directly with the nurse-patient relationship.(19) This situation must, can and will be changed.

However, even the existence of such factors does not justify the daily violation of the patient in those matters that nurses do control. It is not an excuse for the psychological violence to which the person is subjected in the daily living experience as an institutionalized patient. The concept of human advocacy transcends even those situational problems created by physicians who knowingly withhold information from patients because it is based on the patient's humanity and the professional's humanity. This is certainly not a complex concept; rather it is so simplistic that it seems almost ludicrous to propose it. All patients—surgical patients, psychiatric patients, medical patients, pediatric patients, dying patients—are still living human beings with all that this implies. If we remember this—and remember too that we are also human beings—the concept of human advocacy is as natural as living and dying.

ENDNOTES

1. S. Schulman, "Basic Functional Roles in Nursing: Mother Surrogate and Healer," pp. 528–537 in Patients, Physicians and Illness ed. E. Jaco; Glencoe, IL: Free Press, 1958.

2. J. Travelbee, Interpersonal Aspects of Nursing; Philadelphia: David, 1966.

3. Sally Gadow, "Existential Advocacy: Philosophical Foundation for Nursing," paper presented to the four State Consortium on Nursing and the Humanities, Phase I Conference, "Nursing and the Humanities: A Public Dialogue," Farmingham, CT, 11 Nov 77.

4. Leah Curtin, "Nursing Ethics: Theories and Pragmatics," Nursing Forum 17, No. 1 (Spr 78), 4–11.

5. Pierre Teilhard de Chardin, The Phenomenon of Man; NY: Harper & Row, 1959.

6. Feodor Dostoevski, "Notes from Underground," p. 149 in The Short Novels of Dostoevski; NY: Dial, 1945.

7. Rene Dubos, So Human an Animal; NY: Scribner, 1968, p. 40.

8. Gadow, op. cit.

9. Edmund Pellegrino, "A Humanistic Foundation for Medicine," paper presented to the Second International Institute of Health Care, Ethics and Human Values, Mount St. Joseph College, Mount St. Joseph, Ohio, July 76.

10. W.L. Gardiner, Psychology: A Story of a Search; Belmont; CA: Brooks/ Cole, 1970.

11. Rene Descartes, as quoted in Martin Heidegger, Existence and Being; Chicago: Regnery, 1949, pp. 28–29.

12. Richard McCormick, Lecture at Mount St. Joseph's, op. cit.

13. P. Vinogradoff, Collected Papers, vol. 2, ch. 20; Oxford: Clarendon, 1928.

14. Victor E. Frankl, Man's Search for Meaning; NY: Pocket Books, 1963, pp. 160–163. Friederic Nietzsche, The Birth of Tragedy and the Geneology of Morals; Garden City: Doubleday, 1956, p. 299.

15. N. Garver, "What Violence Is," The Nation (June 68), 817–822.

16. Leah Curtin, "Informed Consent: Information or Exploitation?," Update on Ethics 1, No. 4.

17. ANA Code for Nurses, articles 1–3; Kansas City, MO: ANA, 1976

18. Curtin, op. cit.

19. Curtin, "Nursing Practice—A Right and a Duty," Nursing Ethics 1, No. 1 (Fall 78), 7–11.

CHAPTER 5

NURSING ETHICS AND THE ETHICAL NURSE

Myra E. Levine

[Once life and death were in the hands of God. A case shows how a nurse extended human agony for four terrible days—the agony of the dying and the agony of the family. Perhaps it was not moral indifference but mindless use of technology. When did it become immoral to allow someone to die when their time has come? When did it become right to do harm in the name of good?]

To be a nurse requires the willing assumption of ethical responsibility in every dimension of practice. The nurse enters a partnership of human experience where sharing moments in time—some trivial and some dramatic—leaves its mark forever on each participant. The willingness to enter with a patient that predicament which he cannot face alone is an expression of moral responsibility; the quality of the moral commitment is a measure of the nurse's excellence.

It would be flattering to say that our urgent need to face ethical issues in health care has developed out of unusual sensitivity by this generation of health professionals. But it is far more likely that we are a generation frightened by our ability to influence decisions relating to life and death yet, at the same time, unable to fix guidelines for compassion and justice.

In every generation, the caregiver has been well aware of his own vulnerability. Trading on a long tradition of unexamined trust invested in the caregiver by a dependent client, physicians (and nurses, too) have justified the true limitations of their power as a well-disguised secret between the practitioner and his patient. From the days of the cult of Asclepius, the divine gift of the healer has been generally accepted without examination by its bearer, and acknowledged without argument by the patient. The true tilt with fate was clearly a matter between the afflicted and his God, and while not ungrateful for human intermediaries, the outcome was decided by a higher being. It was not difficult, so long as the fiction remained between them, for the practitioner to deal compassionately with his client. The limitations were rarely spelled out but they were almost always understood. Death was a natural phenomenon, easily identified by the cessation of the heartbeat.

But then came the machines which invested in the practitioner the ability to forestall death and even to defy it. It is possible to prolong life, to provide expensive care to some and to choose them over others, to make decisions of living and dying, to make decisions of right and wrong, to mediate issues once forbidden to ordinary mortals. What had been a product of divine will now became a confrontation between people, and the rules which seemed so definitive, no longer comforting or certain.

There must be rules, of course, to govern the relationship between human beings. The rules serve to provide order within the group, but they defend the individuals within it as well. Rules both separate and unite. Their effectiveness depends upon a common acceptance of the guidelines upon which they are based. Within groups that share the same cultural experience, the rules taken together form an etiquette based on the moral basis (the distinction between right and wrong) and is the same for all members. There is, therefore, no need to define explicitly the moral standards upon which the rules are based. The rules of etiquette of one group, however, may not easily transfer to another group which shares a different life experience and depends upon its own code of behavior to regulate it and provide for orderliness.

Where ethical bases of behavior are shared and, therefore, tacitly understood, all parties recognize the rules without further explanation. Armed with such assumptions, the caregiver need not offer extraordinary interpretations of his behavior to the client. In such instances, an unsatisfactory experience may be written off as mere rudeness, abruptness, or a lack of concern—in short, "bad manners." But where the ground rules are in conflict, failure to behave in a "correct" fashion is interpreted as "depersonalization" or "dehumanization" and the argument is raised in the ethical language of right and wrong.

There is small comfort even in the existence of codes of ethics, carefully prepared by a variety of professional groups, since such codes tend to establish rules of etiquette which regulate the behavior of members but are only peripheral to the interests of clients. Indeed, the need to negotiate understanding between groups which possess differing value systems has led to such efforts as publications of the "rights of patients." It is likely that a codification of "rights" will prove no more compelling than the various codifications of "ethics," which superficially influence formal relationships but fail to mediate the informal, one-to-one interactions between caregiver and client that are finally, the most crucial of all. In one hospital, a directive went out to post the American Hospital Association's "*Patient's Bill of Rights*" high enough on the wall to make it difficult to read, suggesting that the institutional commitment was tenuous at best.

Much of the emphasis on ethical issues in health care has been on life and death situations, dealing particularly with the definition of death and the distribution of limited life-sustaining resources. But there are overlooked ethical challenges in the mundane, everyday routine activities of professional practice, and these have gone largely unexamined. Ethical behavior is *not* the display of one's moral rectitude in times of crises. It is the day-by-day expression of one's commitment to other persons and the ways in which human beings relate to one another in their daily interactions.

Every nursing relationship begins with an unusual burden of ethical responsibility. While the patient may have chosen his physician, he does not always have the option of choosing his nurse. The dependency of his patienthood must be based on the assumption that he will be offered care that is, at the very least, effective, and morally responsible.

Responsibility is a factor of the value system which guides the behavior of the nurse, the most basic premise being that the value system of the patient will be recognized, defended, and even cherished. A first step in creating a climate of moral respect essential to a climate of therapeutic effectiveness is to acknowledge that a patient may cling to a system of belief that is different from, and perhaps even contrary to, that of the nurse. Pellegrino emphasizes the importance of this ethical imperative:

"In a matter so personal as health, the imposition of one person's values over another's—even of the physician's over the patient's—is a moral injustice."(1)

While the public media grapple with the large ethical issues of life and death, the range of moral injustices in the daily experience of patients goes on without challenge. There is little in nursing education that prepares the nurse to be a perceptive witness to the moral issues that arise in practice. Until very recently in nursing history, admission to schools of nursing overwhelmingly favored white, middle-class Protestants who fit comfortably into a tradition fostered and protected by the viewpoints of that segment of the population. While the opportunity to enter nursing schools now has broadened considerably, the message of organized nursing thought is still very much that of the white, Protestant ethic, so much so that it is sometimes difficult for nonwhite, non-Protestant nurses to establish effective communication with their peers.

The same limitation of cultural background was a faithful reflection of the populations admitted to medical school so that the "handmaiden" role was not only a consequence of a defined physician-nurse relationship but came quite naturally out of an ethical bias which both physicians and nurses shared. The assumption of surrogate parental roles, in which the physician was the all-knowing father and the nurse the loving, caring mother, left the patient the dependent role of the child who does not know what is good for him. It is a role which unfortunately has persisted and which the patient is expected to play.

The tenacity of that ethical definition is clearly apparent in such groups as those who oppose the Equal Rights Amendment. The ferocity of their battle against encroachment on the comfortable roles established within the old ethical sterotype represents a form of moral injustice rarely equalled. Indeed, if the first level of moral injustice is the failure to acknowledge that other value systems have proper social function, then the next level is the militance with which an individual defends his righteousness as a substitute for acceptance and acknowledgment of another viewpoint.

Self-righteousness is not easily put aside, since it fits so closely the image an individual makes of himself. But self-righteousness is an iron wall between the nurse and the patient. It is in that guise that the patient's diagnosis may establish the entire quality of his relationship with the nurse, bypassing consideration of him as a person.

Diagnostic labels have a life of their own. Some are fashionable and impart to their bearers the characteristics of courage and bravery that demand admiration, while still others suggest profligacy, immorality, and wanton disregard for society's values. There is, for example, tacit recognition that drug misuse and addiction deserve medical attention, but the underlying bias is alive and well every time a postoperative patient is refused prompt narcotic relief from pain on the grounds the he will become addicted. Manipulating the frequency of administration of pain relieving drugs is often rationalized on the premise that narcotic addiction is being prevented. But it is also a consequence of a moral bias that admires the individual who can suffer with stoicism and, thus, prove to his attendants that he is worthy of their efforts in caring for him.

Tight-lipped endurance was associated with the "Yankee" patient in Zborowski's long-outdated study, and it was the Yankee-American who best exemplified the courage and gumption of the brave sufferer.(2) Indeed, the widespread devotion of nurses to that study, for all of its blatant inadequacies, created justification for additional stereotypes beyond those already dear to nursing. Nurse educators wrote texts in which they asked such questions as, "What is the Italian concept of disease?" How gratifying to have a "research" paper to lend legitimacy to an already well-defined moral injustice.

If the stoic is not often among the patient population, then surely the next best candidate for moral approval is the patient who dutifully does only what he is told to do, is undemanding, cooperative, and never, never causes any interference with the orderly routine of the unit. He may be rewarded by being ignored, but that may be an advantage in the long run.

Line reported the struggle of an elderly diabetic woman who made the mistake of begging for additional food and was roundly scolded by the nurses in spite of the fact that she was suffering hypoglycemic episodes every afternoon. Indeed, Line was able to predict from the patient's blood sugars just when the hypoglycemia would occur, and she was convinced that the woman was literally fighting for her life. But a nursing staff who "knew better," and followed meticulously and without question, the established routine, was blinded to the urgent need of that patient.(3) The patient was elderly, diabetic, and spoke with a foreign accent, and each of these factors conspired against her. She was furthermore, a diabetic out of control.

Far too frequently, for all we have learned about the chronicity of diabetes, patients are censured when they reappear with symptoms, because they are believed to have "failed" to take care of themselves. The fiction that diabetes can be controlled absolutely by a therapeutic regimen continues to be attractive to nurses, even though such an assumption is based not on scientific fact but on a moral issue—the specious belief that a diabetic who follows all the rules will live a normal life and that failure is willful.

The same kind of disapproval is often meted out to the smoker, the obese, the elderly, the alcoholic—moral censure that conveys the message that the individual has only himself to blame for the predicament in which he finds himself. There is a disquieting suggestion of this same reasoning in some of the language of the "health-promoters" who ask whether individuals in a society have the "right" to ignore the practice of health measures.(4) Self-righteousness preys on the guilt that always accompanies illness and adds its own weight of shame. How sad that moral censure tells patients they must be grateful whatever the caregiver deigns to give them even at the cost of their own self-respect.

If aggressive defense of one's own value system creates conflict with nursing care needs, then ignorance and indifference to moral issues are even more alarming. The possibility that there is a certain dignity to be found in being criticized rather than being utterly ignored raises moral questions of its own, but there is little doubt that the dehumanizing so deplored in today's care system is based on a view of the individual as an object rather than a person. Perhaps, as Benoliel has pointed out, it is an inevitable consequence of the conditions in which care is provided. She suggests that "social values and structural conditions of work in some settings can be such that providers as well as recipients of care undergo dehumanization."(5) Is it really not possible to provide expert technical care and still retain enough of one's own humanity to recognize and defend it in the patient? The following example raises moral questions for caregivers:

"A dear and close friend had developed symptoms serious enough to warrant an exploratory craniotomy. A deeply devout person, she seemed to sense the grave danger that faced her and went to the operating room resigned and at peace. A tumor so widespread as to be inoperable was found, and she was returned to the intensive care unit in a deep coma from which she would never recover. The surgeon wrote explicit instructions that no extraordinary measures were to be undertaken in the event of respiratory failure. But a few hours after surgery, when her respiration stopped, a nurse standing nearby seized a mask and immediately began to administer oxygen. For four anguishing days, the tragic struggle was continued and, although the family begged the efforts to be terminated, the physician felt he could not then discontinue the respiratory assistance even though he had ordered that it not be used. Finally the equipment was removed. But my friend had wanted her kidneys donated as a gift of life and after four days of assisted respiration, the kidneys proved to be no longer viable. She left us a gift in the blessing her life was for all of us, but she was denied the one last gesture that she had so fervently desired."

It may be unfair to level a charge of moral indifference at the nurse who instinctively turned to the life-prolonging equipment so close at hand, responding automatically to the cue the patient had presented. Still, that nurse dealt with the patient as an object rather than a person. She had failed not only to acknowledge the precise instructions which should have guided her decision in the patient's behalf, but the consequences of her action resulted in four terrible days of suffering for the patient and the several family members and friends who kept vigil at her bedside.

How did it come to be that allowing an individual to die in his time was an immoral act? Indeed, how does one understand the dehumanization of nurses that Benoliel ascribes to their frequent experiences with death in intensive care units? For two decades there has been intense concern with the management of the care of dying patients. After all that time, why haven't we perspective that allows both nurses and the patients their dignity as persons?

So much of our moral responsibility goes unexamined. Nurses are well aware, for example, that the possibility of liability litigation often results in the practice of "defensive" medicine which involves the ordering of unnecessary tests and examinations and even unnecessary or marginally useful therapies in order to protect not the patient but the insurance rate. Indeed, the Hippocratic injunction "to do no harm" has been used to justify a complete range of therapies, all of which are deemed harmless and some of which are equally useless.

The negative command—to do no harm—has been a powerful influence in nursing education as well as in medical education. But, it is reasonable to assume that Hippocrates never intended that it be used for unethical purposes, and any rationalization which excludes the patient's interests as a primary responsibility of health care providers is an unethical one.

Time often changes our understanding of therapy. For example, 20 years ago the level of knowledge made it entirely appropriate to use irradiation as treatment for enlarged tonsils in children. It was impossible to forsee that those youngsters would now be at high risk for the development of thyroid malignancies. So, at that time it was *not* immoral for radiation to be used, but such experiences certainly suggest that only the most exacting criteria should be used to justify care and that the possibility that a therapy will "do no harm" is insufficient.

Nurses once were enjoined to question orders about which they had the slightest doubt. What has happened to that spirit of inquiry? Is it not a matter of moral necessity to call questionable practice to account— whether it be observed in nurses or physicians? Is it not a matter of moral necessity "to do no harm" even when it not possible to do good?

The very nature of nursing makes it impossible for an individual to stand aside from the experience of interacting with other human beings. Nursing has a moral responsibility to be as good as education and self-awareness can make it be. Only intense, personalized involvement can create the moral environment in which care is not only excellent but also a true response to human need. Buber says,

"(He) . . . must stake nothing less than his real wholeness, his concrete self . . . it is not enough for him to stake his self as an *object* of knowledge. He can know the wholeness of the person and through it the wholeness of *man* only when he does not remain an untouched observer. He must enter, completely and in reality, into the act of self-reflection, in order to become aware of human wholeness."(6)

The wholeness which is part of our awareness of ourselves is shared best with others when no act diminishes another person, and no moment of indifference leaves him with less of himself. Every moment of moral injustice exacts a price from both patient and nurse, just as every moment of moral responsibility gives each strength to grow in his wholeness.

ENDNOTES

1. Edmund D. Pellegrino, "Educating the humanist physician: An ancient ideal reconsidered," p. 33 in Fostering Ethical Values During the Education of the Health Professionals; Chicago: University of Illinois and the Society for Health and Human Values, 1976.

2. Mark Zborowski, "Cultural components in response to pain," Journal of Social Issues 8, No. 4 (1952), 16–30.

3. "Insulin reaction in a brittle diabetic: Nursing grand rounds," Nursing (Jenkintown) 2 (May 72), 6–11.

4. American Academy of Nursing, Models for Health Care Delivery: Now and For the Future; Kansas City, MO: The Academy, 1965.

5. Jeanne Q. Benoliel, "The realities of work," in Humanizing Health Care ed. by Jan Howard and Anselm Strauss; NY: Wiley, 1975, p. 182.

6. Martin Buber, Between Man and Man; NY: Macmillan, 1965, p. 124.

SECTION III
NURSING ETHICS AND MEDICAL ETHICS

CHAPTER 6

DEFINING NURSING ETHICS APART FROM MEDICAL ETHICS

Richard T. Hull

[Nursing is concerned with health while medicine focuses on cure. There is a functional difference also in care and healing. The political distinction between nursing ethics and medical ethics is stronger yet. Still none of these alone distinguish the two approaches. Nurses need preparation for the reflective thinking of ethics with or without a difference between medicine and nursing.]

A dean of a major nursing school recently said . . , "We're not interested in *medical* ethics; there is virtually nothing there that is pertinent to nursing. Nursing has its own issues, problems, and principles, and they're quite different from, and often opposed to, those of medicine." She might well have gone on to point out that nursing also has its established codes of ethics and doesn't need a philosopher (especially one who has taught medical ethics), to tell it what is right and wrong, good and bad—but she kindly refrained from that step.

Her comment set me to thinking about the proposition that there is a distinct body of problems, issues and principles for the profession. It seems to me there might be three general arguments to be given in support of this claim, apart from a detailed, nitty-gritty examination of the many facets and dimensions of nursing practice. I shall call these the argument from historical tradition, the functional argument and the political argument.

A. HISTORY

The argument from historical tradition might begin by pointing to Florence Nightingale's 1893 paper. Since then nursing has ascribed to

From *Kansas Nurse,* 55, September 1980, 5, 8, 20–24. Reprinted with permission of the Kansas State Nurses' Association.

the ideals of treating persons rather than diseases. Prevention is better than cure.

Hospitalization has definite limits in its ability to promote "positive health." The history of nursing is a history of nurses' struggles to adhere to these ideals through fostering the patient's active role in treatment and prevention through educational movements, home health care and improved personal hygiene and food handling, and through working for improved hospital conditions to reflect better the psycho-social aspects of illness. By contrast, medicine has opted for an approach that emphasizes curing as a response to the occurrence of disease, a paternalistic approach to medical decision making, and the hospital as the locus of the best medicine.

One might summarize the difference by saying that nursing has conceived itself as a health oriented profession. It emphasizes the preservation and restoration of health to persons. Medicine has conceived of itself as an illness oriented profession. It emphasizes the treatment and prevention of disease, injury and deformity through sophisticated surgical, bio-chemical and technological interventions. Further, nursing has a major preoccupation to compassionately aid individuals to adapt to chronic illness and diminished capacity. Medicine has a major preoccupation with defeating the conditions that make for such diminished lives and capacities. Given such radically different orientations of history and traditions, the argument concludes, it is to be expected that nursing and medicine will have radically different values and ethics.

While there are indeed important differences between some aspects of nursing's and medicine's history, there are some major flaws in the argument from historical tradition. First, a history is always selective and is conceived usually under the guidance of preconceived ideas about the movements and factors one wants to validate historically. Any history is an interpretation which necessarily ignores or discounts as insignificant more than it records.

The foregoing argument ignores the close ties between the ideals and aims of nursing and medicine that have been commonplace for decades before and since Nightingale. It ignores the preventive and wholistic movements in medicine. It ignores the specialization and compartmentalization in nursing against which the total patient care movement was a reaction. But most importantly, a historical argument does not establish anything but a description of (some) past practices and patterns. In and of itself, it does not establish any authority for their preference and continuation at the present. The description may be accurate. It does not form a sound basis for the generalization that there are and should remain important differences between nursing and medical ethics.

B. FUNCTION

By contrast, the functional argument proceeds from a description of present nursing practices and a theoretical account of what nursing should be ideally. The actual details of the history of nursing and medicine may not demonstrate the divergence of their ethics and values. If one looks at function and if one subsumes present practice under nursing theory, one can see the difference that supports a different ethic.

For example, in contemporary practice, the typical physician interaction with a patient is brief. It is to get a medical history, symptoms and signs, consent to a proposed intervention, or compliance. All this serves the goal of cure. The physician reviews examination and test results, arrives at a diagnosis and therapeutic regimen. S/he writes orders, supervises specialists in administering therapeutic procedures, and checks on the patient's progress. By contrast, the nurse's interaction with patients is much more extensive and personal. It focuses on the patient's values and perceptions and adaptive/restorative processes. Nurses may have been co-opted as physician's assistants. Yet nursing ideally functions not as an extension of the physician but as a complement.

A root metaphor is sometimes used, although its sexist overtones make it unfashionable among more politically minded nurses. Nursing has affinities with the maternal functions of nurturing, education and caring for the young. The term derives from the Latin "nutrio" meaning to nurture. Thus nursing is like ideal mothering. It fosters education, growth and protection of those in child like states where they are unable to provide for their own nurture. Medicine, by contrast, is not focused on nurture of health, but on combat with the enemies of health—disease, malfunction and injury. The root Latin here is "medicus," healing or making whole again. The language of medicine reveals the process is thought of in warlike terms: combat, struggle, defeat, fighting are commonplace. The functional understanding of medicine is struggle against an enemy. The nurse and the physician are primitive mother and father, nurturing children and protecting them from the enemy. The functional argument concludes the ethics are different. Compassion and support are fundamental virtues in nursing. Courage, authority and risk taking are those of medicine.

Important as these functions are, to insist that they are specially tied to nursing and medicine is to caricaturize, not characterize, these professions. The recognition of the essential integration of healing and nurture has waxed and waned periodically in medicine and nursing both. But in the ideal functioning of those arts, they are inseparable. The recurrent interest in wholistic medicine, preventive medicine and family practice, public sanitation, diet therapy and psychosomatic medicine are all responses of medical professionals. They perceive that the best medicine integrates nutritive and disease combative functions rather than treating them as independent and inseparable. Nursing is moving towards informing and improving its functions with more formal training. It is increasingly active in history taking, physical examination, diagnosis, and technical therapy. Specializations are emerging like anesthesiology, intensive care and pediatric practitioners. This points to a recognition that there is an essential connection between the supportive and diagnostic/therapeutic modes of involvement with patients.

Thus, the most that the functional argument can hope to establish is that there is a difference in emphasis in nursing and medicine. But that reflects more a division of labor from specialization of training than divergences in fundamental underlying processes and concerns of the professions. Certainly one cannot point to the ideal of each profession and say, "Here are clear differences that must manifest themselves in different ethics." Both professions share a commitment to the health and well-being of individuals. There is a commitment to defeat disease, to marshall all the person's psycho-social resources, as well as physiology, to use modern medicine in defense and comfort of the ill and infirm. Here are grounds for mutual ethical commitments by both professions, rather than a different ethic.

I will return to this line of argument shortly. It is first desirable, however, to consider the political argument for the view that nursing and medicine have different ethics.

C. POLITICS

This turns on a class or economic struggle between nursing and medicine. Those engaged in the struggle, see nursing as having served too long in medicine's shadow. They believe that nurses have inadequate working conditions, pay and public respect. For nurses to get these, nursing must be defined as an independent profession. It must get away from the maid servant image. Nursing must organize and even unionize to get economic leverage and the power to dictate better working conditions. Such developments as independent nurse practitioners much be encouraged to gain public respect. So nursing must be defined as independent. That includes the area of ethics. Nursing ethics ought to be articulated to reinforce nursing's independence of the profession of medicine.

Functional differences do not serve the purpose. The nurturing, maternal figure does not accord with economic independence and enhanced status. That tradition has reinforced the subservient posture. Attention to language also means new terms so that patients become clients. There is a conscious effort to avoid sexism—feminine pronouns for nurses and masculine for physicians. There is a national movement to the baccalaureate degree for nursing. Doctoral programs have been designed in nursing as opposed to the traditional routes for doctorates in education and communication.

I am ambivalent toward the political argument. Nurses have received the short end of the economic stick. They have not been given public respect and the status they deserve. They have been exploited in work. At the same time, I find it alarming as a consumer of health services, that the conclusion is drawn so easily that nursing ethics is different from medical ethics.

To say that nursing ethics is wholly different from medical ethics would imply that the principles of conduct, moral aims and obligations of nurses and physicians differ even in the same sets of circumstances. Further, it would imply that those professionals would be under no positive obligation to coordinate their actions [unless their ethics called for coordination as in the ANA Code for Nurses]. One ethic might dictate the patient be told the exact nature of the illness while the other said no. Both could not be done. The outcome would lie with whichever professional had the clout to dominate.

Finally, on this political basis, one could justify a separate ethic for any health care profession—physical therapists, hospital administrators, etc. Any group would have a right to define an independent ethics. Nor would nursing itself be assured of unity. Nurse anesthetists function differently from nurse practitioners and may have differing political needs. LPN's and LVN's might find it politically expedient to organize in contradistinction to RN's. Each of these political facts and functional differences could, if the earlier lines of argument held, result in a separate set of ethical commitments [unless, again, the ethics called for coordination].

The proponent of the political argument could say reality means compromise on differences. This could mean developing a consistent interprofessional set of ethical principles. Politics sees money as basic. Politics is the art of the possible. So the give and take of the bargaining table might well be the proper method for resolving differences. Such bargaining would not ensure the best interests of the consumer. So the consumer might be a party to such negotiations.

There are other concerns. Without a set of common assumptions and commitments as a basis for resolving issues, the resolution may be based on political and economic power. Nurses will lose—particularly with the medical profession actively creating new health professionals who are taking over nursing functions while staying under more direct control by physicians. (That's a political argument against the political argument!)

Moreover, there is a deep-rooted relativism underlying the political argument which at bottom is absurd. How can it be sensible to say that what a patient has a right to differs according to whether a physician or nurse is involved? A physician is obligated to get informed consent before proceeding with a risky invasive procedure. How could it make sense that the nurse who administers it is not under an obligation to stop if the patient does not understand? How can it make sense to say a physician can refuse to do an abortion but the nurse can't? A particular level of education may determine professional privileges but not moral rights and duties. If it did, it would be moral elitism that flies in the face of universal moral rights and obligations.

How effective the foregoing argument is against the view that there is an independent nursing ethics, I cannot judge. It is quite possible that nursing, or substantial factions within it, will remained committed to a political approach. But perhaps it would be worth while to explore a set of common ethical principles for a common basis for new relationships with medicine.

But there are still questions if such an inquiry is needed and who will make it? At the beginning I mentioned another line of objection that might be taken to the intrusion of a philosopher in nursing ethics. This hints at a number of points which need to be laid out more fully.

Nursing has several codes of ethics: The International Council of Nurses' "Code for Nurses" (rev. 1973), the American Nurses' Association "Code for Nurses with Interpretive Statements" (rev. 1976; Statements rev. 1985), various other countries and provinces and some nursing specialties. Nurses who take the Florence Nightingale Pledge ascribe to a set of ethical ideals there as well. Finally, specific institutions have their own rules and standards of conduct. Nurses do not lack ethical standards. Do they need anything more?

Skill in applying such rules requires reflection. What are the options? Who decides? How is the decision made? A code gives guidance but it may be ambiguous. Rules may conflict as in research. A nurse contributes to the profession's body of knowledge by research. However, a research protocol may require a placebo as a control and that may include deception. To decide which rule to follow and which to violate, the nurse must appeal to a broader set of principles. That may mean setting priorities.

No code has ever covered all ethical dilemmas. The view that all a nurse needs is a code, is oblivious to this [and does not understand the nature of the code]. The unwary may believe they do not have to grapple with decision making that involves more than applying a rule. Finally, while a great deal of careful thought went into the codes, that very fact indicates they are not immune to criticism or improvement. Technology has increased our choices. Nurses are taking increased responsibility and independence. The professions will be better served by active critical discussion to improve the codes than to pretend they are beyond changing. (This is not to say there are no timeless ethical truths. Rather, particular statements of them may be relative.)

The other part of the criticism referred to earlier involves an alleged breach of professional integrity. The argument may go like this: unless also qualified as a nurse, a philosopher has no business being critically involved in discussions of nursing. Everyone has had bad experiences with busybodies, moral do-gooders who charge in to set aright situations where their arrogance is exceeded only by their ignorance. The non-nurse ethicist is in grave danger of being just such a busybody.

This is an ironical view since nursing has many criticisms of medicine, etc. There are, of course, important differences since nurses know medical procedures while a non-nurse philosopher does not. Beyond additional training, perhaps the philosopher can only point to the results and wear the scarlet letter when the title of busybody has been earned. But there is additional justification for critical examination.

Philosophical training helps one wear different hats to generate the best possible reasons for conflicting views. A philosopher should be able to present systematically, sympathetically and forcefully the viewpoints of others in a dispute. It may be difficult to pin a philosopher down on his/her personal convictions. Steve Martin, the comedian, calls this a kind of permanent confusion from the study of philosophy. More important, it is the conviction that fairminded, intelligent people can disagree on pretty fundamental issues. Such disagreements are less the result of personal stubbornness than differences in traditions and culture. It takes time and reflection to see the bases of such disagreements, and possibly to resolve them. This is especially true in ethics where questions have been called perennial and where concepts have been said to be essentially arguable.

The philosopher has acquired some comfort in dealing with these questions and concepts. On this basis, s/he can discuss them with other professionals, rather than speaking as a true believer out to reform the world. A dilemma may disappear when looked at carefully. Sometimes a decision made elsewhere will already have answered a troublesome question in a new area. Sometimes an issue involves a very basic choice between competing principles. One's very foundations may be shaken and reformed by that choice. Should any of these experiences occur, the discussion will be considered worthwhile.

FOR FURTHER READING

Elsie L. Bandman and Bertram Bandman, Nursing Ethics in the Life Span; Norwalk, CT: Appleton-Century-Crofts [A-C-C], 1985.

Leah Curtin and M. Josephine Flaherty, Nursing Ethics: Theories and Pragmatics; Bowie, MD: Brady, 1982.

Joy Curtis and Martin Benjamin, Ethics in Nursing; NY: Oxford, 1981.

Ann J. Davis and Janelle C. Kreuger, Patients, Nurses, Ethics; NY: AJN, 1980.

Lucie Y. Kelly, Dimensions of Professional Nursing; St. Louis: Mosby, 1981.

Catherine P. Murphy and Howard Hunter, Ethical Problems in the Nurse-Patient Relationship; Boston: Allyn & Bacon, 1983.

Joyce E. Thompson and Henry O. Thompson, Bioethical Decision Making for Nurses; Norwalk, CT: Appleton-Century-Crofts, 1985, p. 7.

————, Ethics in Nursing; NY: Macmillan, 1981.

CHAPTER 7

CONFLICTING LOYALTIES OF NURSES WORKING IN BUREAUCRATIC SETTINGS

Joyce E. Thompson

INTRODUCTION

The reality of the practice of nursing today is that more than 80 percent of registered nurses are hired to carry out their professional duties by someone other than clients or patients. Nurses are employees. Another reality in the practice sphere of nursing is that more than 75 percent of nurses are employed in hospital settings, often very large bureaucratic institutions with their own sets of rules and obligations. So while subscribing to an idealized role in the health and illness care of others,(1) nurses are often thwarted in their attempts to practice professional nursing by the very institutions that purport to assist them in the health and illness caregiving functions.

This paper will explore the multiple duties and obligations of nurses as professionals who are also employees in bureaucratic institutions that have their own loyalties and obligations. I will begin with some definitions of terms so that you can better understand my reasoning process as this paper develops. Next, I will identify some of the major sources of conflict and moral dilemmas for nurses who work in hospital settings, including some case studies for illustration and analysis. Finally, I will close with a summary of the major conflicting work obligations and loyalties for nurses in today's practice world.

CASE

I had the pleasure of assisting in the birth of the infant son of Tom and Jane in a large tertiary care center in the Northeast. As the baby was

Reprinted with permission from *Professionalism and the Empowerment of Nursing*, American Nurses' Association, Kansas City, Mo., pp. 27–37, copyright 1982.

born healthy and quietly into the eager hands of one of my midwifery students, I asked the mother if she would like to hold her son right away. Her response was instantaneous: "Is it all right?" The nurse in the room started to object, but I gently and firmly said, "Of course; he's your son!" The mother immediately reached between her legs to grab hold of this new person and accepted him gently onto her bosom. A warm blanket was placed over infant and mother, and Tom was invited to help dry his son. Three times during the next 15 minutes the nurse asked if she could have the baby so she could weigh him, put the silver nitrate in the eyes, and take his footprints, and three times the mother said "not yet," supported each time by the midwife. Later, when I questioned the nurse about her reasons for wanting the baby right after birth, she answered that she was new to the setting and did not want to go against hospital policies. She admitted she didn't know what those policies were yet. She had not attended a birth with a midwife before, and didn't know we were allowed to give babies directly to the mother when they were born. She thought they had to go to the warmer for heat and suctioning.

My internal response to this brief conversation was a "My Word! What has happened to our nursing commitment of meeting patients' needs with caring and sound clinical judgment when we resort to use of hospital policy as our sole basis for decision making?" I could not contain myself, so I asked, "Whose baby is it? Did you think he was cold? Did he need suctioning?" We continued our discussion about balancing patient needs with nursing judgment, but we were interrupted by the head nurse asking for help with another patient. Someday I hope that nurse and I will finish our discussion.

Commentary

These are some of the questions I would like to raise with her. How is it that childbearing women have to ask if it's all right to hold their own baby? What has happened to hospital oriented childbirth that it is forcing some couples to choose out-of hospital care or no care at all, rather than submit their bodies and normal life experiences to the control of others—doctors, midwives, nurses? Have nurses lost so much control over their practice in hospitals that they can no longer use humanistic clinical judgment in making decisions? Who makes hospital policies and for whose benefit are these policies made? The hospital? The nurses? Or the patient?

I have deliberately chosen this case study to illustrate the pervading, day-to-day, insidious, and potentially harmful state of nursing practice in many of our hospitals today. This situation is all too common. It is not the headline story of the moral dilemma in termination of life support for a Karen Quinlan. And, I propose that because it is not the subject of headlines, because it rarely gets discussed openly, such a situation is an even more ominous symptom of potentially unhealthful nursing practices in institutional settings.

I propose to begin and open a hopefully productive dialogue on nursing: its practice, its conflicts, its obligations, duties, and loyalties. Addressing myself both to those who have reflected on the ethical and legal rights, duties, and obligations of nurses and to those who have not, I suggest that it is imperative that nurses examine their daily nursing practices, looking particularly at the ethical dimensions of their decision making in health and illness care. If nurses are to live up to their status as professionals, they must practice in an ethical manner, and this means studying ethics in order to determine what is ethical practice. As noted earlier, the particular focus of this paper will be on the ethical and moral dilemmas of nurses who are employees in hospital settings.

Some of the questions I would ask each nurse employed by a hospital include: "When was the last time you stopped to ask yourself whether you did your best today on behalf of your client or patient? If you were kept from doing what you thought should have been done, what or who provided the obstacle? Do you think your hospital's policies are essential for patient care? How many times today did you stop to determine if an act of nursing care was in accord with the physician's plan of care or hospital policy, or ethical practice for the patient you were assigned? Were all of your nursing actions based on reasoned decision making, or were some of them routine, without thought of their appropriateness to the particular person you were caring for? If you had the day to do over again, would you change any of your nursing actions? Why? Would you consider an alternative plan of action or care for Mrs. Jones? or Mrs. Smith? or baby Tom? Did you finish work today with a sense of peace or a gnawing discontent, unsure of where the bad feelings were coming from?"

These questions are only a few examples of critical self-examination of one's professional practice. They may, by pointing to sources of conflict, lead to increased understanding of the ethical and moral dimensions of nursing practice. Before examining the sources of conflict for nurses who work in bureaucratic settings, it is appropriate to define some terms to provide a common basis for discussion.

DEFINITIONS

In our work in ethics and nursing, my husband and I have found it helpful to distinguish between the terms "ethics" and "morals," even though they have a common root in Greek and Latin.(2) We define morals as the "shoulds and oughts" of life, and ethics as the reasons, the "whys" behind the morals. The earlier questions raised the moral "should" for your examination, such as, *should* nurses use hospital policies to decide how to care for patients, or should all patients be treated with respect and dignity? The ethical dimension asks, "why"? What is the basis for treating patients with respect and dignity? What is the ethical principle used to support the "rightness" of hospital policy? Ethical principles usually examined include autonomy, beneficence, nonmalficence, justice, and veracity.

In keeping with the writing of Lucie Kelly(3) and Smith and Davis,(4) I believe that as one enters a profession (such as nursing), there are certain rights, duties, and obligations that one assumes. Many authors find it helpful to distinguish the ethical from the legal. For example, Smith and Davis define a legal right as a "claim recognized as valid by the legal system" and an ethical right as a "claim called for by ethical principles or an enlightened conscience and not necessarily by legal rules." Similarly, duties flow from one's role status, legal ones as defined in the law and ethical ones as required by ethical principles. A legal obligation is incurred by a contract, whereas an ethical obligation is incurred by a relationship based on a commitment.

It should be obvious from this brief discussion that nurses as professionals have both legal and ethical rights, duties, and obligations that at times may be quite similar and at other times are distinct and even in conflict. In fact, as has been noted by several authors,(5) nursing actions can be both ethical and legal, or ethical yet judged illegal, or quite legal but unethical—depending on the ethical framework used to judge the action. The *ANA Code for Nurses*(6) defines many ethical duties and obligations. These include the duty of providing nursing services with respect for human dignity and the uniqueness of the client; safeguarding the client's right to privacy; protecting clients and the public from the incompetent, unethical, or illegal practice of any person; assuming responsibility and accountability for nursing actions and judgments, and maintaining competence. The Code also mentions duties to the profession of nursing and other health care efforts. Keeping in mind that there are both ethical and legal duties and obligations, and that often these are different, it is reasonable to expect these may be in conflict at times. If one expands the notion of ethical duty or obligation to include the concept of loyalty, the chances for conflicting claims on the nurse's time and efforts increase. The concept of loyalty (as distinct from duty or obligation) comes from within the individual nurses as she chooses to whom her loyalty will be given at a specific time or in a given situation, and on what basis. This loyalty may coincide with the nurse's legal obligations or her ethical obligations, or it may be based on friendship or other human factors.

SOURCES OF ETHICAL CONFLICT

With these definitions in mind, I will now focus on some of the sources of ethical conflict in bureaucratic settings. There are at least four major sources of conflicting obligations and loyalties: (1) the setting or institution, (2) the other players on the team, (3) the nurse's employee status, and (4) the nurse's personal ignorance of the ethical dimensions of practice and the ethical reasoning process. I will examine each of these sources of conflict in some detail in seeking the reasons why some nurses experience work dissatisfaction or·unexplained discontent in hospital settings (ethical conflict) and others do not.

The Bureaucratic Institution

Anne Davis,(7) Catherine Murphy,(8) and others (9) speak often of the social context within which nurses practice and make decisions in health and illness care. The very nature of hospitals as large bureaucracies implies a hierarchical order of employee status. Many nurses could quickly define where they think they are in the bureaucratic pecking order and relate that position to what they should do. For example, they might feel that the bureaucracy often discourages or ignores criticism, supposedly in the best interests of the whole "family."

The ethical theory subscribed to by most hospitals is that of utilitarianism, often summarized by the phrase "the greatest good for the greatest number." At present I will ignore the problems of who defines the "greatest good" or who are the "greatest number," and focus briefly on how the utilitarian position in health care can cause major conflicts for nurses (and other health care workers who believe in and provide care based on deontological (principled) concern for the individual client. For example, if one were to use the principle of justice to judge actions, is it *just* to require all babies to return to the nursery during visiting hours even if no visitors are expected and a breast-fed baby is hungry? Is there value in promoting efficiency of staff functioning to the detriment of individualized patient care activities? How do you explain what has happened to some nurses in the past who have taken an ethical stance by defying hospital policy in the interests of the patient, by reporting incompetent practices of a colleague, or by refusing to carry out a physician's order which was deemed not to be in the best interests of the client, and subsequently been dismissed from their job, put on a graveyard shift, or otherwise harassed by co-workers and administrators? One might question the ethical basis for these latter actions.

Another example of potential conflict inherent in large hospital settings has been the increasing development and use of technological aids in caring for patients. Technology has created choices most nurses didn't dream about in nursing school. And even when nurses learn *how* to use the machine, they don't often learn the equally important concept of *when* to use such technology. What should the response be when it appears that certain technology is over-used in order to recoup the original financial investment from third party payers of clients who don't really need the test or machinery?

Likewise, it is interesting to note that what is now considered ordinary medical treatment in large hospitals is still extraordinary in smaller facilities, and especially so for some clients, who may even deny that I.V. fluids are ordinary measures to take in certain human conditions. Who should make the decisions on when to use technology, and on what basis should such decisions be made? Do nurses inadvertently support the abuse of technology because they don't take the time to question whether a patient really needs the procedure? Ignorance is no excuse for avoiding conflicts in bureaucratic settings. Likewise, it is important periodically to ask whether we are nursing the patients or the hospital. What are the values and virtues of the hospital we work in and are they consistent with good care for patients? Are these practices consistent with ethical practice of professionals?

The Players

Other sources of potential conflict of obligations and loyalties for the nurse in the hospital are the various players on the health/illness care team. These players include the patient, physicians, other nurses, auxiliary personnel, administrators and business manager, the patient's family, the social worker and society, and others. It seems logical that the individual nurse can easily receive conflicting demands (claims) for loyalty and service from each or all of these players, often simultaneously.

We enter into relationships with each or all of them in any one day, and their needs can be quite different.

Probably the most easily recognized ethical conflict is that posed when physician and patient disagree on the treatment plan and the nurse is asked to take sides. The physician may expect support based on the nurse's obligation or loyalty to him as captain of the team, while the patient expects patient loyalty and nursing duty will determine the nurse's choices.

For some nurses this conflict never arises, because they accepted a support-the-physician role early in their careers and have lost the sense of critical inquiry needed to base each act of loyalty on the merits of the specific situation. Likewise, some nurses avoid the conflicting loyalties between patient and health care institution by deciding their job is essential and so their primary commitment is to their employer—the person paying their salary.

Probably one of the most frustrating situations of conflicting obligations for nurses is the situation of a patient who refuses to participate actively in decisions about his care or who seemingly is uninterested in regaining his health. After all, how can the nurse carry out her ethical obligation to support self-determination of clients when the client doesn't want to be autonomous? Lowenthal(10) notes that a person who is ill wants help, not autonomy; but that does not absolve the nurse of the obligation to treat patients with respect and human dignity. Helping may not always be best for a given individual or his state of health, however. My favorite example of such potential conflict is a New York teen clinic that provided model team care for pregnant teenagers. As the nurse-midwife director began to note an increased recitivism rate (repeat pregnancies), she asked why. The response was that the teens had never had such loving care and attention, and they had to be pregnant to get it. The staff quickly decided to start a parenting program for these teens. Caring can create the very situation we are working to prevent.

Employee Status

As noted earlier, nurses as hospital employees are placed in a hierarchical network of power. They carry multiple responsibilities to patients, employer, and co-workers; and demands from any one of these may conflict with both ethical and legal obligations to the others. Because of their relatively low power status in the bureaucracy, nurses have often been called upon to carry out decisions made by others (physicians or patients) without benefit of participating in the process and understanding why such a decision was ordered. This is a very difficult situation to be in, and can potentially result in poor care for assigned clients.

When we enter into a relationship with clients by virtue of our membership on the health care team (in contrast to physicians, who may be contracted with directly), we may be obligated to care for clients we would not have chosen if we had made the original contract. Some authors suggest that this very fact of coming along with the "package" of health and illness care places the nurse in a unique position of being obligated to carry out Statement One of the *ANA Code for Nurses*—respect for human dignity and the uniqueness of clients—even when we may disagree personally or professionally with their reasons for being in the hospital or the manner they choose to deal with their health problems. I suggest that nurse-patient relationships are based on a covenant of a responsive and promissory state of commitment to provide needed services and in return require active participation from the client in working towards health. William May(11) is quick to note that covenant fidelity to the patient remains unrealized if it does not include proficiency as well as humaneness. Likewise our ANA Code speaks to our duty to retain competence in nursing as well as to care for assigned clients.

It is in this arena of assignment of patients that legal and ethical duties may come into conflicts as well. The commitment to care for certain clients, whether personally opposed to their choice of activities such as euthanasia, needs to be balanced with the legal and ethical duty not to abandon clients. The situation of conflict may be avoided if there are other staff present who can accept the assignment the nurse disagrees with. However, if no one else is available to care for this client, I suggest the moral duty to provide care and not abandon is more pressing than the right to refuse to care on personal grounds. In my ethics work with various health professionals, values clarification seems to help professionals know themselves well enough to begin to anticipate patient care situations of potential conflict, and therefore choose employment or assignments that will minimize their chances for personal-professional turmoil, rather than finding themselves in the middle of a situation that becomes intolerable for both nurse and patient. While few of us have such freedom of choice in where we are going to work, I question whether the fact of "forced" employment diminishes one's ethical and legal obligations to clients assigned for care. Does the personal situation of needing employment wherever one can find it lessen the responsibility to practice in an ethical manner? We have already discussed how some nurses choose work patterns by loyalty to institution and physician over patient or self, so maybe they can also choose not to be in turmoil over personal beliefs.

The Nurse Herself

The final area of potential conflict for nurses who are hospital employees is that between oneself and one's personal beliefs and the professional commitment to provide nursing services in an ethical manner. When I ponder why some nurses are not in control of their practice, I keep returning to the idea that it is because they choose (consciously or unconsciously) to not be in control! You may think this a harsh accusation against my colleagues; but the more I work in nursing and with various levels of pre-professional and professional students, the more convinced I am of the importance of deciding for oneself whether to be in control of nursing or to let others control one's practice. There are many people waiting and willing to take over control of nursing practice should nurses choose to give up their autonomy!

FURTHER CONSIDERATIONS

In spite of the fact that I have discussed at length the nature of the hospital setting, the variety of nurse relationships in bureaucracies, and employee status as potential sources of conflicting obligations and loyalties for nurses, I do not give these as reasons for less than ethical nursing practice. These conflicts make it more difficult for some to carry out their nursing responsibilities at times, but they certainly should not be used as excuses for poor or unethical nursing.

One of the major reasons nurses compromise their caregiving activities and provide less than optimum services to clients and employers is ignorance of the ethical dimensions of practice and ethical reasoning in conflict situations. Many nurses have not had formal preparation in these topics during their nursing program or in continuing education programs. Many do not even know that the *ANA Code for Nurses* exists, or what it says regarding the ethical duties and obligations of those who call themselves nurses.

To be sure, most nurses recognize the signs of cognitive dissonance (conflict) as they practice, but many ignore the symptoms or choose to follow directions of other, more powerful team members (physician, administrators). Without the tools to work through moral dilemmas in nursing practice, some nurses have chosen paths of least resistance: avoidance of a particular patient or physician with whom they sense disagreement, calling in sick when they anticipate an unfavorable work assignment, deferring all decisions to "the doctor," blaming the institution for the inability to make decisions or act autonomously, and, if the conflict seems too big to handle, quitting that job and looking for another. The irony and sadness of these types of behavior is that moral reasoning erodes if not used, and patient care slips with it.

Those who have attempted to take an ethical stance in their work setting with little support from colleagues or employer know how difficult it sometimes is to reason morally and to act ethically. Lucie Kelly(12) in an editorial in *Nursing Outlook* wrote of the nurse's dilemma in ensuring informed consent. She noted that it is easy to pontificate about the nurse's ethical and legal responsibilities, but why is patient advocacy relegated to "maverick, martyr, or team player?" I suggest that one of the major reasons that ethical stances in nursing practice are not always supported by colleagues is the fear associated with supporting change or a position not in keeping with the powerful: the institution or the physician or the patient. The reality is that nurses probably lose their jobs for taking an ethical stance more often than for incompetent practice.

Mila Aroskar(13) asked whether nurses have the mind set to practice ethically. Who we are as nurses is based on who we are as persons (our values and beliefs) as well as how we perceive our role in health and illness care. Nurses relate with a variety of people in their daily work settings and have many demands on their time. What they do to handle these demands will determine the quality of nursing practice. Hence the question, do nurses have the mind set to practice ethically?

SUMMARY

There is a choice in nursing. Nurses can choose to practice ethical nursing which requires understanding and action, including ethical inquiry, principled thinking, strategies for action, and a spirit of compassion for oneself and for others.(14) Or they can yield, as many of their colleagues have done in the past, to the utilitarian, sometimes unethical demands of hospital employers, with the excuse that it is not worth the battle or that they cannot do anything as one person, or that they do not want to be a martyr.

Nurses have a choice, both individually and collectively. To be professional is to be ethical.(15) To be ethical is to be autonomous. Nurses need to maintain or gain (or regain) control over their own practice and their profession if they truly care what happens to their patients. Good nursing care that promotes self-actualization and autonomy and wellness in patients will be impossible unless nurses are in positions of control of what and how they do nursing. The ultimate authority to care for a patient comes from the patient.(16) How nurses care is their responsibility.

ENDNOTES

1. Catherine P. Murphy, "Models of the Nurse-Patient Relationship," pp. 8–24 in *Ethical Problems in the Nurse-Patient Relationship* ed. Catherine P. Murphy and Howard Hunter; Boston: Allyn Bacon, 1982.

2. Joyce Thompson and Henry O. Thompson, *Ethics in Nursing;* NY: Macmillan, 1981.

3. Lucie Y. Kelly, *Dimensions of Professional Nursing;* NY: Macmillan, 1981.

4. Sharon J. Smith and Anne J. Davis, "Ethical Dilemmas: Conflict among Rights, Duties and Obligations," pp. 6–20, this volume.

5. Thompson and Thompson, op. cit. Mila A. Aroskar, "Anatomy of an Ethical Dilemma," this volume.

6. American Nurses' Association, *Code for Nurses with Interpretive Statements;* Kansas City, MO: ANA, 1976.

7. Anne J. Davis, "Social Role Constraints on Ethical Decision-Making by Nurses," pp. 160–164 in *Nursing Law and Ethics;* NY: Springer-Verlag, 1985.

8. Catherine P. Murphy, "Making Clinical Judgments: From a Nurse's Point of View," in *Making Clinical Judgments* ed. Clem Davidson; Carbondale, Illinois: Southern Illinois University, 1982.

9. Aroskar, op. cit. Myra Levine, "Nursing Ethics and the Ethical Nurse" this volume. Larry Churchill, "Ethical Issues of a Profession in Transition," AJN 77, No. 5 (May 77), 873–875. Paula Sigman, "Ethical Choice in Nursing," ANS 1, No. 3 (1979), 37–52.

10. Uri Lowenthal, "Medical Care: The Problem of Autonomy," pp. 28–38 in Carmi and Schneider, op. cit.

11. William F. May, "Code, Covenant, Contract, or Philanthropy," HCR 5, No. 6 (Dec 75), 29–38.

12. Lucie Y. Kelly, "Neither Maverick nor Martyr," NO 2, No. 8 (Oct 80), 644.

13. MIla Aroskar, "Are Nurses' Mind Sets Compatible with Ethical Practice?" *Topics in Clinical Nursing* 4, No. 1 (Ap 82), 22–32.

14. Thompson and Thompson, op. cit.

15. Churchill, op. cit.

FOR FURTHER READING

Mila Aroskar, "Are Nurses' Mind Sets Compatible with Ethical Practice?," Topics in Clinical Nursing 4, No. 1 (Ap 82), 22–23.

———, "Ethics of Nurse-Patient Relationships," Nurse Educator (Mar–Ap 80), 18–20.

Elsie L. Bandman and Bertram Bandman, "The Nurse's Role in Protecting the Patient's Right to Live or Die," ANS 1, No. 3 (Ap 79), 21–35.

Bertram Bandman, "Do Nurses Have Rights? No," AJN 78 (Jan 78), 84–86.

Elsie L. Bandman, "Do Nurses Have Rights? Yes," AJN 78 (Jan 78), 84–86.

———, "How Much Dare You Tell Your Patient?," RN 41 (Aug 78), 38–41.

M.E. Carnegie, "The Patient's Bill of Rights and the Nurse," Nursing Clinics of North America 9 (Sep 74), 557–562.

Barbara A. Carper, "The Ethics of Caring," ANS 1, No. 3 (1979), 11–19.

C.M. Chapman, "The Rights and Responsibilities of Nurses and Patients," Journal of Advanced Nursing 5 (Mar 80), 127–134.

Anne J. Davis, "Dilemmas in Practice: To Tell or Not," AJN 81 (Jan 81), 156–158.

Willard Gaylin, "Patient Rights, Nursing Responsibilities," Nursing Digest 1 (Oct 73), 5–8.

Lucie Y. Kelly, "Nurse, Will You Tell?," NO 26 (Feb 78), 135.

P. Sigman, "Ethical Choice in Nursing," ANS 1 (Ap 79), 37–52.

K.M. Sward, "The Code for Nurses: Historical Perspective," pp. 1–9 in Perspectives on the Code for Nurses; Kansas City, MO: ANA, 1978.

Joyce E. Thompson, "Conflicting Loyalties of Nurses Working in Bureaucratic Settings," pp. 27–37 in Professionalism and the Empowerment of Nursing; Kansas City, MO: ANA, 1982.

CHAPTER 8

NURSING ETHICS, PHYSICIAN ETHICS, AND MEDICAL ETHICS

Robert M. Veatch

[Nursing ethics is a legitimate but very limited subcategory of medical ethics. Physician ethics is a very powerful subcategory. In the health care team, neither are captain of the ship. Both should begin with the patient.]

The term "nursing ethics" is controversial. Some insist that nursing ethics is a unique field posing issues that cannot be understood fully by adapting the professional ethics of physicians. They insist that the term "nursing ethics" connotes the uniqueness of the moral problems that nurses face in the health care setting.

On the other hand, others argue against the term. Some suggest that it is demeaning and has somewhat the connotation of watered-down ethics—the flavor of such textbook titles as *Anatomy For Nurses* or *Pharmacology For Nurses*. Others critical of the term "nursing ethics" argue that there is really very little that is morally unique to nursing. The same ethical principles and the same moral issues emerge in the health care setting whether one is a physician, nurse or patient.

This article puts forth the view that nursing ethics is a legitimate, if very limited, term referring to a field that is a subcategory of medical ethics [or, better, of health care ethics—see later (eds.)].

MEDICAL ETHICS

Medicine is a sphere of human activity dealing with the well-being of the body. Medical ethics is simply the ethics of decisions made within the medical sphere. Most such decisions are not made by health profession-

Reprinted with permission from *Law, Medicine & Health Care*, vol. 9, no. 5; copyright 1981, American Society of Law & Medicine, Boston, Mass.

als, either nurses or physicians; they are made by lay people facing problems in the medical sphere. When an individual lay person decides to take an aspirin for a headache, he or she makes a medical decision. When a parent examines his small child's wound and decides not to take the child to the emergency room, he makes a medical decision. When Congress decides to increase or restrict Medicaid coverage, it makes a medical decision, that is, a decision in the medical sphere, by allocating medical resources. Medical decisions only rarely involve consultation with health care professionals. All medical decisions must be rooted in some general system or theory of ethics. That ethical foundation may be grounded in a religious tradition, a secular world view, or an explicitly articulated normative ethical theory. A set of values, however, is expressed in any such decision. To the extent that the values are ethical, it can be said that a decision incorporates a judgement in the medical sphere, or, for short, medical ethics.

Some small fraction of these decisions is made by medical professionals—people who earn their livelihoods by working in the medical sphere. Among this small fraction made by medical professionals, an even smaller portion is made by physicians. The analysis of the ethical decisions made by physicians can be called physician ethics. It is a subcategory of the large field of medical ethics. Reasonably, physician ethics would be derived from that same general system of ethics that provides the foundation for all medical ethics. This is not to argue that there are no special moral obligations for physicians—of course there are. But those special duties should make sense in the context of a more general ethical framework and should, in principle, be acknowledged by anyone adopting that framework. Reasonable people should be able to deduce an ethical framework that they want physicians to apply in medical judgements within the physicians' sphere.

Similarly, nurses make some of the professional medical judgements. The analysis of ethical decisions made by nurses can be called nursing ethics. Like physician ethics, it is also a subsystem derived from a larger general system of medical ethics.

Physician ethics and nursing ethics are sometimes articulated by those standing in a religious tradition or a general secular tradition. On some occasions, however, the professionals within each group articulate their own conception of their duties. We might call this a professionally articulated ethic or simply, a professional ethic. Thus, there may be professional physician ethics or professional nursing ethics, distinct from physician ethics or nursing ethics.

Presumably, both the nurse and the physician ground their own articulations of their duties in a more general system of ethics. Within this general system, special duties may be deduced for people in special professional roles. Whether these special "role-specified" duties are articulated from inside or outside the profession, the same general moral theory should apply to physicians, nurses and all other medical decision makers, including the lay people who make most of the medical decisions in any culture.

THE ISSUE OF POWER: PHYSICIAN ETHICS VS. NURSING ETHICS

The question remains whether there is any difference between physician ethics and nursing ethics and, if there are any differences, whether these are related to differences in roles. It could be that the difference between physician and nursing ethics is based in the professions' different subject matters. For example, the nursing role is sometimes erroneously viewed by some members of society as being passive and as following orders. Yet, this view is inaccurate. For example, if a terminally ill patient were receiving an intravenous antibiotic, holders of this view might say that the physician could appropriately decide that the IV should be stopped, while the nurse would only follow orders and stop the IV. If that were the case, then physician ethics would include an elaborate framework for the ethics of deciding to stop antibiotics on terminally ill patients, while nursing ethics would be relegated to some simple ethic of following orders. However, this seems wrong on two counts.

First, it can be argued that it is always wrong for a physician to decide on his own to stop medical treatment. The decision to continue or stop medical treatments must be made by patients or their agents. The physician's moral dilemma is actually quite different, since he must decide whether to collaborate in other continuing care when the patient or the agent has decided to end certain life-prolonging treatment. Perhaps the physician also faces the question of whether to intervene physically to provide the undesired life-prolonging treatment as an act of civil disobedience against the wishes of the patient. The moral problem of the physician is secondary or subsidiary, however, to that of the patient as primary decision-maker.

Second, it is equally wrong to conceive of the nurse as one who simply follows orders and removes the IV without moral reflection. In reality, the moral question for the nurse is the same as that for the physician: whether to collaborate in other continuing care when the patient or agent has decided to stop certain treatments.

Thus, the subject matter of physician ethics and nursing ethics, at least in the above example, is the same. In fact, there is no area where the subject matter of the two ethics differs. Members of both professional groups must decide whether to participate in abortions, whether a consent is adequate to justify touching a patient, whether they should give patients information, or whether they can justifiably disclose confidential information to others.

If there is a difference between nursing ethics and physician ethics at all, it is a difference in role relations of the two professions. One moral problem for any ethical theory is what an individual's moral obligations are when the person feels an act is wrong, but that act has been ordered by someone else. Nurses often face this problem. They are placed in positions of power deficit where the ethics of carrying out ordered acts become a dominant ethical theme.

In contrast, physicians are typically in positions of power. Their ethical problem has not been one of power deficit, but of power surplus—the ethics of abuse of power and authority. Physicians must ask themselves such questions as: "Even though I know I can get a patient to behave in a certain way, is it morally appropriate for me to use my power and authority to get such behavior?"

Recently, however, this traditional balance of physicians' power surplus and nurses' power deficit has begun to change. As medicine is practiced more and more in organized, institutionalized, and structured settings, physicians are increasingly part of a health bureaucracy. Less and less the isolated individual practitioner is found in that romantic stereotype of the one-to-one patient-physician relationship. Physicians are part of a medical service; they are members of a department or at least part of a group practice. Their work is supervised by Professional Standards Review Organizations (PSROs) and Health Systems Agencies (HSAs) and subject to state and federal regulations. So, physicians are increasingly faced with the problem of the ethics of the power deficit. They must decide whether to engage in civilly disobedient acts of falsifying Medicaid records in order to get reimbursement to which they are entitled. They must decide whether to refuse to follow the instructions of the department head or the senior attending physician. Moreover, if the physician's role becomes one of a convenantal relationship with an active, thinking patient who makes medical decisions, the physician will have to place moral constraints on the free exercise of the power and authority that has traditionally been vested in his role.

At the same time the nurse is emerging as an independent practitioner. Nurses are now functioning in the role of nurse-practitioner, primary nurse, clinical nurse specialist, counselor, or nurse-midwife. In these new roles, nurses formulate treatment plans and act substantially as independent agents. If there is a difference between nursing ethics and physician ethics over questions of power and authority, it is at most one of degree, with nurses more frequently and more realistically facing the problems of being expected to engage in practices that violate their own consciences, while physicians frequently act from positions of relative moral autonomy. Both perspectives, however, emerge at least upon occasion in both professional fields. In the teaching of ethics in health professional settings the situation is, unfortunately, still such that it is prudent and pragmatic to give more emphasis on this moral problem of power deficit when one is teaching nurses than when one is teaching physicians. Unfortunately, more nurses than physicians find themselves in situations where they must decide whether to carry out ordered acts to which they morally object. The difference, however, is one of emphasis. In principle, the problem of power deficit and power excess can be faced by either professional group.

THE HEALTH CARE TEAM

It has been suggested that the nurse inherently occupies a different position in the health care team than the physician. The emergence of the concept of the health care team suggests new kinds of moral considerations, such as the duty to consult and to collaborate with colleagues. It might be that different positions on the team lead to different role-related duties. A hospital-based nurse, for instance, finds it impossible to provide more than about one-fourth of the nursing time for the hospitalized patient, whereas virtually all of the physician contact may come through or at least be supervised by one individual. It might be argued therefore that the nurse is inherently more a part of the team and that the ethics of "team play" separates nursing ethics from physician ethics.

That the two play different roles on the team cannot be denied. But once again the physician is increasingly part of the team and is part of a collegial group of physicians providing the physician care. The physician is also interacting as part of the broader health care team. It could be argued that the physician is the captain of the team, while the nurse is only a player on the team. The seems unacceptable, however, for a number of reasons. Each has a limited sphere of responsibility and independent decision-making authority, but neither is really the captain of the team, or at least neither really should be, since it is the patient around whom the team is organized and to whom the team is dedicated. It makes sense to view the patient as the captain of the team. If that is the case, then the team ethics do not differentiate physician ethics and nursing ethics. Thus, differences in role relations do not provide an account of differences between nursing ethics and physician ethics any more than do differences in subject matter or differences in the foundation of norms.

HEALTH PROFESSIONAL ETHICS

Professional nursing ethics is by definition different from professional physician ethics. One is articulated by nursing professionals while the other is articulated by physician professionals. That, however, seems to be a very minor technical, historical or sociological difference between the two. When we turn to more general conceptions of nursing ethics and physician ethics that are not necessarily articulated by the professional groups but are rooted in a common moral framework, the two seem to have even less significant differences. Both nursing and physician ethics deal with ethical problems of role relationships, including relationships to the health care team. They deal with a common subject matter and are both appropriately viewed as deriving moral obligations for their specific roles from a more general or universal system of medical ethics that physicians and nurses alike share with patients in the medical community.

Thus, nursing ethics and physician ethics may be different only to the extent that the same ethical framework is being applied to the same kinds of issues in two different professional groups. This is only a linguistic or analytical difference. Both kinds of ethics might more appropriately be called health professional ethics. Health professional ethics in turn might be seen as a branch of a larger field called medical ethics that provides a general moral framework and which includes normative reflection on the medical decisions made by both lay persons and professionals.

The role of the nurse is not identical to that of the physician. It is inappropriate to use the concept of medical ethics which views the physician as primary decision-maker or to apply the concept of the exclusive, isolated patient-physician relationship to the context of nursing. These routes are inappropriate, however, not because the nurse's ethical position is any different from the physician's. Rather, it is wrong to view any health professional as a primary decision-maker for patients and to maintain an image of any health care professional as existing in an exclusive, isolated patient professional relationship. The differences between nursing ethics and physician ethics then may not really be that great. They especially will not be if the articulation of the ethical framework for both professional roles begins with the patient as the primary active agent and decision-maker.

FOR FURTHER READING

J.A. Ashley, Hospitals, Paternalism, and the Role of the Nurse; NY: Columbia, 1976.

Elsie L. Bandman and Bertram Bandman, Bioethics and Human Rights; Boston: Little, Brown, 1978.

Vincent Barry, Moral Aspects of Health Care; Belmont, CA: Wadsworth, 1982. [One of the few balanced approaches that consider nurses as well as physicians and other health care professionals]

Alexander V. Campbell, Moral Dilemmas in Medicine: A Coursebook in Ethics for Doctors and Nurses, 2nd ed; Edinburgh: Churchill Livingstone, 1975.

Eric J. Cassell, The Healer's Art: A New Approach to the Doctor-Patient Relationship; Philadelphia: Lippincott, 1976. [Cassell treats patients rather than diseases. eds.]

Anne J. Davis and Mila A. Aroskar, Ethical Dilemmas and Nursing Practice, 2nd ed; NY: A-C-C, 1983.

G.F. Donnelly, A. Mengel, D.C. Sutterly, The Nursing System: Issues, Ethics, and Politics; NY: Wiley, 1980.

Barbara Ehrenreich and D. English, Witches, Midwives, and Nurses—A History of Women Healers, 2nd ed.; Old Westbury, NY: Feminist Press, 1973.

M.J. Fromer, Ethical Issues in Health Care; St. Louis: Mosby, 1981.

Lucie Y. Kelly, Dimensions of Professional Nursing, 4th ed; NY: Macmillan, 1981, Ch. 13; "Professional Ethics and Accountability."

Edward D. Pellegrino, "Educating the Humanist Physician," Journal of the American Medical Association 227, No. 11 (18 Mar 74), 1288–1294.

R.B. Purtillo and C.K. Cassell, Ethical Dimensions in the Health Professions; Philadelphia: Saunders, 1981.

Robert M. Veatch, Case Studies in Medical Ethics; Cambridge, MA: Harvard, 1977.

SECTION IV
DECISIONS AND DECISION MAKING

CHAPTER 9

PLURALISTIC ETHICAL DECISION MAKING

Rita J. Payton

[Ethical theory in bioethics tends to focus on deontological ethics and utilitarian ethics. Nurses are not normally absolute deontologists or utilitarians. The author offers a model for decision making composed of both.]

ETHICAL THEORY

Three ways of thinking that relate to morality and ethics are discussed by Frankena.(1) The three approaches are considered different study traditions of ethics. The first tradition or way of thinking about ethics is called descriptive ethics. A descriptive ethicist is one who is concerned with how people actually behave. The goal is to describe and explore the phenomenon of ethics that is actually present in a given situation.

The second tradition of ethical thinking is called normative ethics. The normative ethicist asks what is right, what is good, or what is obligatory. The normative ethicist is concerned with the rationale for action and with an appraisal of the decision-making process that occurred before the action was taken. The normative ethicist must be ready to give reasons for his judgement about action; in other words, he is concerned with the process of justification.

The third study tradition of ethics is concerned with metaethical thinking. Metaethics is basically concerned with the semantics of meaning and is sometimes described as analytical thinking. Metaethics is not concerned with action decisions in particular situations. Rather, it is concerned with answers relating to logic and semantics.

Davis and Aroskar believe that the study tradition of normative ethics

---

Reprinted from Clinical and Scientific Sessions, American Nurses' Association, 1979. Used with permission.

is the tradition most useful in a program of study in bioethics for a professional nursing curriculum.(2) The professional nurse must often debate with self or with someone else about what is good or right in a particular patient concern or as a general principle. The latter type of thinking relates most directly to the normative ethics study tradition.

An ethicist is one who is engaged in an ongoing critical reflection on morality. A critical reflection on morality can take place at several levels of discourse, discourse with one's self or with another. Four levels of ethical discourse are discussed by Aiken: (a) particular judgement, (b) moral rules, (c) moral principles and values, and (d) reasons for being moral.(3) The level, moral principles and values, and the level, reasons for being moral, are more useful for professional nurses as they justify their decisions.

DEONTOLOGICAL ETHICS

Normative ethics is considered as comprising two major schools, the school of deontological ethics and the school of teleological ethics. Deontological ethics, or the ethics of formalism, recognizes the existence of prima facie duties or obligations. Such duties include the fulfillment of promises, the payment of debts, and the telling of truth. Such duties admit of no exception regardless of the circumstances in a particular situation. The deontological system holds tha tthe rightness of an act is either not entirely determined by the value of its consequences or is not at all determined by the value of the consequences. The basic principle of deontological ethics is that the ethical act does not entirely depend on the consequences of the action. Rather, the ethical act is that act which is in agreement with one's duties and/or obligations.

In order to know whether an act is right or wrong, one needs to determine whether it is in accordance with a valid moral rule. Ross believed that the rightness of an act may in part be determined by the goodness of its consequences, but that it is never wholly determined by such good consequences.(4) Deontological ethics maintains that there are duties or obligations affecting action that have moral validity independent of the consequences of individual actions. One must act in accordance with these duties and obligations.

The principle of universalizability means that an action principle or duty obliges everyone without exception. Another important principle of an action principle or duty is that it is necessary. The word necessary means that the rightness or wrongness of the action has no relation to the nature of the world in which the doer finds her/himself.

TELEOLOGICAL ETHICS

Teleological ethics judges an action as either morally right or wrong by judging the consequences of the action, according to Brody.(5) Teleological ethics is also called consequentialist ethics. The teleological ethicist denies that the nature of the action itself is either morally right or morally wrong. Rather, the consequences of the action alone determine the moral worth of the action. The teleologist's primary objection to deontology is the idea that obligation or duty can in any way be self-evident. If duty or obligation is self-evident, then how are we to explain irresoluble differences of opinion about what ought to be done? The rise of the teleological ethical school came about primarily in response to this objection to deontology.

Utilitarianism is that form of teleological ethics that utilizes the single ultimate principle. In other words, utilitarian ethics is a kind of consequentialist ethics. Utilitarian ethics is the largest branch of ethical theory within the teleological school of ethics. The utilitarian single exceptionless principle is that the right action is that action which produces the greatest amount of pleasure or good for the greatest number.

The major assumption that separates teleological ethics from deontological ethics is that moral issues can be determined by empirical calculation. One can weigh the value of a given consequence or combination of consequences against a different consequence or combination of consequences.

In the teleological ethical system, moral significance is always future oriented. In other word, no moral significance can come from historical duty or obligation. In discussing teleological utilitarianism, it must be emphasized that the standard of value for judging must be both impartial and universalizable.(6) Impartiality is best viewed as the fact that everyone counts as an equal unit of one. Universalizability is the assumption that everyone in similar circumstances would do the same act.

Rawls viewed the structure of an ethical theory as basically determined by how it defines and connects the notions of the right and the good.(7) The right refers to the nature of the action itself, and the good refers to the consequences of the action. The simplest way of relating the two basic notions is taken by teleological theories; the consequences are defined independently from the action, and then the action is defined as that which maximizes the desired consequences.

BIOETHICAL PLURALISM

Very few, if any, professional nurses make decisions according to either pure deontological ethical reasoning or pure teleological ethical reasoning. In everyday, realistic situations, people are concerned with both the means and the ends of their actions. Means of action can be conceptualized as the "right" or the nature of the action. The ends or consequences of the action can be viewed as the "good", the "good" that results from the action.

Does the professional nurse originally isolate the ethical thought process on means rather than ends, or on ends rather than means? As most people in real situations do when faced with a need to make an ethical decision, professional nurses are concerned with both means and ends simultaneously. Bioethical pluralism refers to the simultaneous concern with both means and ends. Bioethical pluralism denies that the morality of an action is determined either by consideration of the means of the actions alone or by consideration of the ends of the action alone.

Bioethical pluralism is a term preferred by this writer as more useful in describing the actual ethical system in use by most professional nurses. The pluralistic ethical system is not teleological in nature, nor is it considered truly deontological.

ETHICAL DECISION MAKING

Professional nurses are constantly and deeply involved in situations requiring ethical decision making. Dependence on the American Nurses' Association's professional code for nurses alone will not provide nurses ethical answers in specific patient care situations.(8) Therefore, professional nurses must develop the skills necessary to make personal ethical decisions in relation to their professional role.

Broad social and cultural changes have affected nursing structures and decision-making processes. Dominant political scenes now include human rights and individual autonomy. Pluralism and personal freedom are highly espoused. At the same time, there has been an increase in bureaucratization and development of complex social institutions to deal with public problems. The complex health care delivery system is an example.

The content of the concept of bioethics is vital and dynamic, because morality cannot be identified without some reference to the context of action. This writer denies an absolute fact-value distinction. The expansion of knowledge from rapid technological advancement influences moral decisions. Knowledge increases our choice options, and moral or ethical behavior reflects choice options. Fact is always changing as our knowledge base changes. What was moral at one point in our history of understanding could now be immoral because of a change in our base of knowledge. One result of this latter viewpoint is that fact and value are

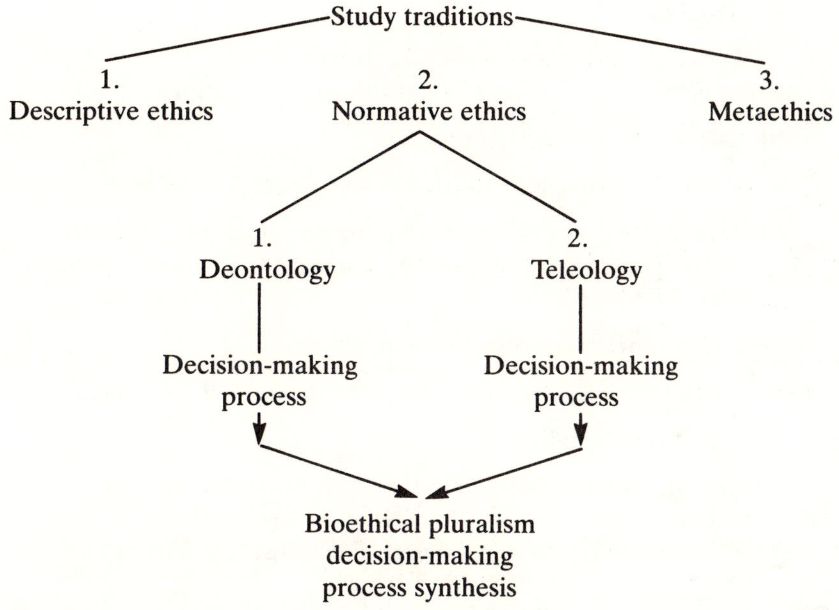

Figure 9.1 Theoretical conceptual framework for deriving pluralistic decision-making model.

part of morality and, therefore, we cannot hope to find exceptionless and absolute rules of morality. It has become essential that professional nurses develop skills and a comfort level with an ethical decision-making process that will be useful over a span of time regardless of the changes in the knowledge base upon which they function.

Some basic questions arise as one attempts to define a useful pluralistic decision-making model. The first question explores whether a rational decision-making process that is powerful enough to determine priority in the face of conflicting value interests actually does exist. The second question concerns the possibility of establishing such a reasonable decision-making process by rational methods of inquiry. The purpose of normative ethics is to use inductive and deductive logic to arrive at reasonable ethical action decisions.

PLURALISTIC ETHICAL DECISION-MAKING MODEL

Brody developed two distinct ethical decision-making processes, the first for the teleological ethicist and the second for the deontological

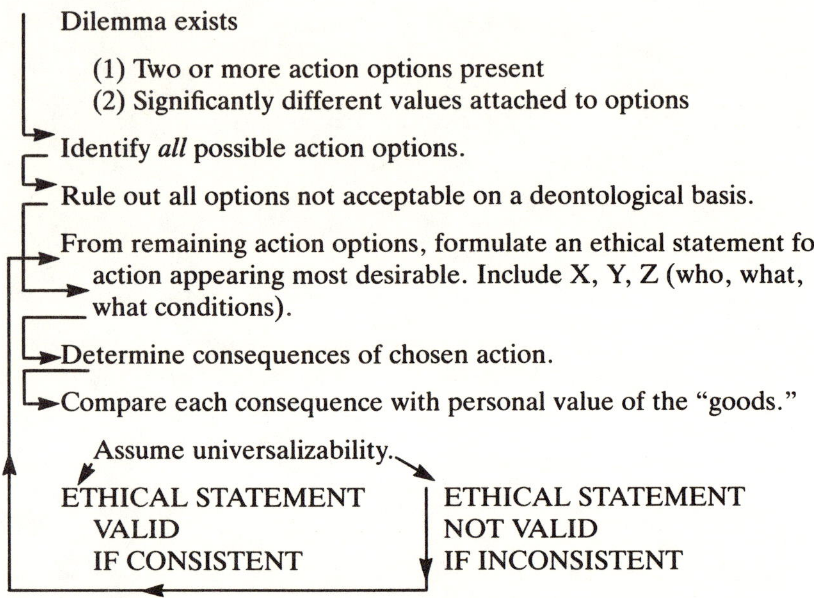

On cycle return in case of invalid result:

(1) Ethical statement may be reformulated modifying the
conditions.
(2) Alternatie action option (still available after rule in) may be
explored going through all remaining steps.
Remember: the decision to take no action is in itself action.

Figure 9.2 Pluralistic ethical decision-making model. An original synthesis of the deontological and teleological decision-making models of Brody.

ethicist.(9) His models are simple, clear, and concise. They therefore possess characteristics that are essential for a model if that model is to be useful for the professional nurse. As this writer has expressed earlier, however, practicing nurses do not seem to reason in a pure deontological manner or in a pure teleological manner. My work represents a synthesis of Brody's original models. The synthesis should be more useful for the professional nurse because it allows for simultaneous concern with the nature of the action and the consequences of the action.

Some basic skills are needed before one engages in ethical decision making, regardless of the decision-making model utilized. The most obvious skill is recognition of an ethical dilemma when it exists. Inherent in this skill is the ability to separate true ethical or moral dilemmas from dilemmas that are really nonethical or nonmoral. Power and/or authority struggles are often labeled ethical dilemmas; so are technical differences of opinion.

Potential ethical dilemmas for the nurse have to be analyzed for the presence of at least two variables. The first variable relates to the number of action options truly available to the nurse. If it is truly only possible for the nurse to take one action, then no dilemma exists. More than one real action option must exist before an ethical dilemma can be said to exist. The action option that is most frequently overlooked is the option to take no action. Taking no action whatsoever is often a very powerful action option and must never be forgotten.

The second variable that must be analyzed when determining whether or not an ethical dilemma exists is the value weighting the nurse would give to the consequences flowing from the various action possibilities. If the combined consequences of action A have a weighted value equal to the combined consequences of action B, and so forth, than it is doubtful whether a true ethical dilemma exists. For example, when two nurses have differing opinions about how best to position a patient for a given procedure and no scientific basis exists for defending one opinion over the other, it is very doubtful whether an ethical dilemma exists. A power struggle or dilemma may ensue, but an ethical dilemma is just not present.

Once it has been determined that an ethical dilemma does in fact exist, the nurse proceeds to make a list of all possible action options. It is rare when only two actions are possible. Every attempt should be made to make the list of action options exhaustive. Often a third or fourth option will prove more useful than the first two possible actions occurring to the nurse. Often we cut off our thinking after coming up with two action options and carry on an either-or type of struggle.(10)

The nurse now needs to compare each action to her set of *a priori* moral principles or rules. These rules exist because of predetermined duties or obligations. The nurse who has difficulty determining her own *a priori* ethical rules could probably benefit from various clarification strategies, which are so popular today. As one example, the action option in a given patient situation might involve the nurse giving the patient a truly lethal dose of a medication. However, the nurse recognizes and accepts an *a priori* principle that states that one may never kill except in self-defense. This particular nurse would, therefore, have to rule out the action option that would require the giving of a lethal dose of a medication. Each listed action option must be screened through the individual's own list of predetermined moral or ethical rules. Those action options that violate individual moral rules or principles must be eliminated.

At this point in processing the dilemma, one action option will seem to stand out as the most desirable. It would seem only reasonable to acknowledge this human response. So the nurse should choose the most desirable appearing action option and formulate a moral statement. The ability to formulate a moral statement is a skill that requires understanding of the principle of universalizability. A formula for a moral statement is this: "In situation X, person Y ought to do thing Z."(11)

The nurse ought not administer a preoperative medication to a patient who has not expressed informed consent for the proposed surgical procedure. This looks like a fairly adequate ethical or moral statement. The nurse is Y, administering the preoperative medication is Z, and the rest of the statement seems to be X. But the conditions X are really not complete. We do not expect infants or incompetent adults to give informed consent. Therefore, the moral statement would have to be modified by perhaps inserting the words competent adult in place of the word patient.

The principle of universalizability would mean that all nurses ought not administer preoperative medication to any competent adult who has not expressed informed consent. The nurse cannot put the personal self "I" into an ethical statement. This would violate the principle of universalizability and reduce the statement to a statement of personal opinion contingent upon the circumstances of the time.

The next step of the decision-making process is to determine and list all the possible consequences if everyone were to follow the proposed ethical statement. It is important that both immediate and long-term consequences be defined. We all tend to be concerned mainly with the immediate consequences and tend to forget to explore the ramifications for the future. It is probably humanly impossible to define all consequences, but we should attempt to "reduce uncertainty to manageable proportions."(12) Undoubtedly, 10 years from now when one looks back at ethical statements that one has formulated, some will appear obsolete or untrue. That does not mean the statement was not valid when it was formulated. It is an indication of the reality that the body of knowledge upon which ethical judgements are made will change with the passage of time. As the facts as we know them change, so may our ethical determinations change.

Once one has determined all possible consequences to the best of one's ability, it is time to proceed to the next step of the decision-making process. Each of the consequences must be compared with the individual's value set. Once again, it is imperative that nurses individually develop insight into the relevant health care related values of their total value set. Since the nursing profession is inherently a human-to-human interaction, a large proportion of an individual's total value set is relevant. Values relating to autonomy, paternalism, truth telling, justice, and confidentiality are just a few of the relevant values. Values clarification techniques again might prove useful in aiding individual nurses in gaining the needed insight.

If the possible consequences do not seriously violate the personal value set, the proposed ethical statement will be congruent or valid and the individual should feel free to take action as contained in the ethical statement.

It is very common for one or more of the consequences to come into conflict to some degree with the value set. When this happens, the ethical statement is considered incongruent or invalid. There are two basic methods to utilize when incongruence occurs. The ethical statement may be tightened up by modifying or clarifying the conditions, X, in the statement. If modification of the statement cannot eliminate major incongruences, then it may be necessary to choose another action option. When a different action option is chosen, it must itself be processed through all the remaining steps of the decision-making model.

The pluralistic decision-making model will obviously not guarantee consensus among members of a nursing or health care team. But consensus probability is certainly greater than with a process that involves the simplistic sharing of opinions and feelings about what ought to be done in a given patient situation. The individual nurse, furthermore, emerges knowing much more about his or her personal value set and can contribute much more at a rational level in ethical decision making.

ENDNOTES

1. William K. Frankena, Ethics; Englewood Cliffs, NJ: Prentice-Hall, 1973.

2. Ann J. Davis and Myra A. Aroskar, Ethical Dilemmas and Nursing Practice; 2nd ed.; Norwalk, CT: Appleton-Century-Crofts, 1983.

3. Henry D. Aiken, Reason and Conduct: New Bearings in Moral Philosophy; NY: Alfred A. Knopf, 1962.

4. W. David Ross, The Right and the Good; Oxford: Clarendon Press, 1930.

5. Howard Brody, Ethical Decisions in Medicine; Boston: Little Brown, 1976.

6. P. Taylor, Principles of Ethics: An Introduction; Encino, CA: Dickenson Publishing Co., 1975.

7. John Rawls, A Theory of Justice; Cambridge, MA: Belknap Press, 1971.

8. American Nurses Association. Code for Nurses with Interpretative Statement; Kansas City, MO: The Association, 1976.

9. Brody, op cit., p. 11, A-2a.
10. Ibid., p. 9.
11. Ibid. p. 6.
12. Ibid. p. 10.

CHAPTER 10

ANATOMY OF AN ETHICAL DILEMMA

Mila A. Aroskar

[An ethical dilemma has a theoretical and a practical component. The author analyzes the structure of a dilemma in terms of ethical theory, decision theory, time, and a data base. This serves as a framework for the analysis of an actual case.]

Examination of the anatomy of ethical dilemmas within health care generally, and specifically in nursing, is an essential first step in the thoughtful consideration of dilemmas. Ethical dilemmas occur both at the nurse-patient-family level of interaction in hospital and home settings and at the policymaking level of institutions and communities.

Ethical dilemmas have always been with us, but their nature in health care settings has changed radically with the development of new knowledge and technology. Years ago, nursing texts addressed such "ethical" concerns as appropriate behavior between physicians and nurses, respectful wearing of the uniform, and the need for nurses to follow the ethical policies of the hospital. In the 1980s, this does not even touch on the complex ethical dilemmas faced by both individual nurses practicing in bureaucracies and by the nursing profession itself.

Bioethics, as a discipline applying ethical thinking to the health sciences, has developed most rapidly within the last decade. Traditionally, ethics has had to do with individual decisions regarding what should be sought in life and what should be avoided, ways and goals of life, and duties and obligations. Bioethics concerns choices and conflict around such health care issues as longevity versus freedom from pain, full versus partial disclosure of health information, rights of individuals versus rights of society, and rights among individuals in the distribution of limited health care resources.

How does one begin to think about and structure these complex issues which involve so much uncertainty and ambiguity?

A.   ETHICAL THEORIES

Ethical theories and reasoning do not solve ethical dilemmas. They do suggest ways of structuring and clarifying them. They help us go beyond slogans.

We can look at what three positions in ethical reasoning—utilitarianism, egoism, and formalism or deontology—offer in the way of suggested solutions. Each position structures ethical dilemmas in particular ways.

Utilitarianism

At the present time, the utilitarian position prevails in looking at many ethical dilemmas in delivery of health care to individuals and society. It focuses on consequences of actions, on the greatest amount of happiness or the least amount of harm for the greatest number . . .

Egoism

If one takes the egoistic position, one seeks the solution that is best for oneself. The nurse acting within an egoism framework would consider the solution that is most comfortable for him or her without regard to the benefits and harm to the patient, family, or any others. The solution may or may not be beneficial to the patient; however, the patient is not the primary consideration.

Formalism

In the formalist or deontological position, one would look neither at one's own personal position nor at the consequences of actions. Instead, one would consider the nature of the act itself and the principles or rules involved; never tell a lie; do unto others as you would have others do unto you, and so forth. Immanuel Kant is considered to be in the formalist tradition with his "categorical imperative" that one should act on a maxim which one can apply in any similar situation(1)—the principle of universalizability. One often hears a mother invoking this concept when she says to a misbehaving child, "What if everyone did what you're doing?" Another version of this imperative is that persons should always be treated as ends, never simply as means. In the recent past, people have been used as means in some research.

Fairness

Another position for consideration is presented by John Rawls, an important contemporary theorist on justice. Rawls talks about justice as fairness. According to his thinking, distribution on burdens and benefits should be considered from the point of the least advantaged in society; for exmaple, children or the poor should share the benefits in society equally with all others. Benefit to the least advantaged becomes the norm for decision and policy making.

Rawls suggests that in considering the validity of moral principles one must look at the following:

Universality: Principles must apply to everyone, and one must take into account the consequences if everyone complies.
Generality: Principles must apply widely and not refer only to specific people or situations.
Publicity: Principles must be publicly recognized by everyone involved.
Finality: Moral principle is the final court of appeal and overrides the demands of law and custom on the basis of principle.(2)

These criteria rule out all forms of egoistic position from the moral point of view.

B.   STRUCTURE OF A DILEMMA

The process of structuring an ethical dilemma for purposes of clarification, decision, and ultimately, action may take a variety of forms. One way that I have found useful in working with nursing groups is to break the dilemma into three elements—situational "facts", decision-making questions, and underlying ethical theories—and to view these elements within the context of time and value systems. (See Fig. 10.1.)

To clarify the elements, one must:

1. Elucidate the data base that one needs in order to do moral inquiry.
2. Consider the questions that come from decision theories.
3. Articulate the moral approaches, positions, or theories to be used in considering alternative action.

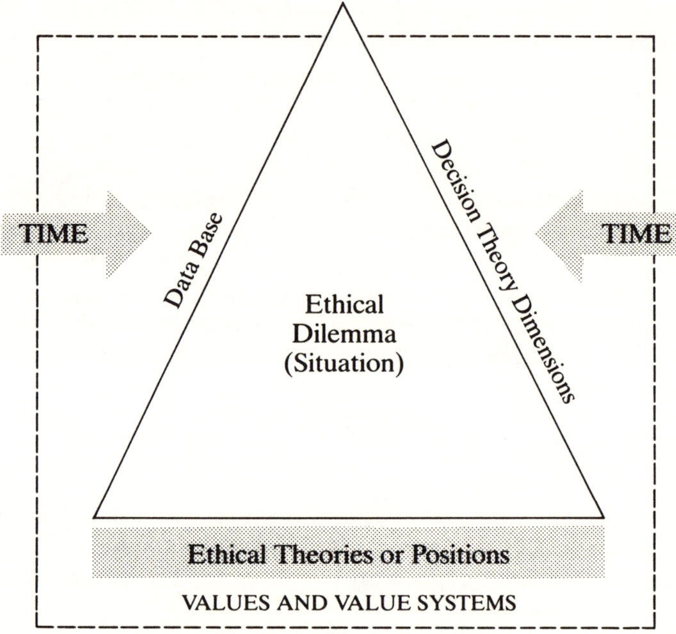

Figure 10.1 Dimensions of an ethical dilemma.

Value systems

The personal and professional value systems of the decision makers and of those affected by the decision will, of course, underlie the above three elements. For example, one person may consider that death is the worst that can happen to an individual, whereas another person involved in the same situation may feel that a severely handicapped life is a worse alternative when there is a choice to be made. Other values that may be involved in dilemmas for the nurse are those related to obedience and following physician orders, use of coercion to achieve certain ends, and the importance of patient self-determination.

Time

This is yet another dimension in clarifying dilemmas. Some dilemmas demand immediate action. Those in which time is less critical offer more opportunity for evaluating information as well as identifying and weighing options prior to action.

Data Base

To examine an ethical dilemma, first of all one has to identify whether an ethical dilemma exists—especially when the dilemma is not as obvious as, for example, switching off a life support machine. Then, to gather the data base for ethical inquiry, the following questions should be answered as completely as possible:

1. Who are the actors involved? What are their histories and involvement in the situation?
2. What is the proposed action or actions?
3. What is the setting or context of the proposed action?
4. What is the intention or purpose of the proposed action?
5. What other alternatives or choices are available?
6. What are the probable implications or consequences of the proposed action?

This is different from the data base that nurses are accustomed to gathering, but it contains such familiar concepts as assessment, and it extends the reflective thinking process to an identified ethical dilemma. One may not have all the data available that one wishes to have in decision making. However, decisions often must be made without the ideal data base in the real world. Furthermore, even though the data base provides an essential component in consideration of an ethical dilemma, decisions do not simply spring from heaps of data.

The second element of the triad for structuring an ethical dilemma is to consider the following questions which come from decision-making theories:

1. Who should decide? The physician, nurse, patient, family, committee? Why?
2. For whom is the decision being made? Self, proxy, other?
3. What criteria should be used? Social, legal, physiological, economic, psychological, other? Why?
4. What degree of consent by the client or subject is needed? Freely given, coerced, none?
5. What, if any, moral principles are enhanced or negated by a proposed course of action? Self-determination, truthfulness, beneficence, justice as fairness?

In thinking about these questions, nurses and nursing students should also examine the concept of paternalism, or maternalism, as the case may be. When is the nurse interfering with a person's liberty and autonomy for the good of that individual in order to force what he or she, the health professional, considers to be a reasonable choice? When, if ever, do considerations for social good override the rights of the individual to make his own decisions about health care? These decisions may be easier in such situations as an epidemic of communicable disease where the community is clearly in danger. But they become particularly difficult and ambiguous when children, the mentally ill, or others determined to be incapable of decision making are involved: for example, in alleged child abuse situations or commitment of the mentally ill.

Ethical Theory

The third part of the triad in structuring an ethical dilemma is to begin to articulate ethical theories or positions in looking at alternatives for action in a specific situation.

The decision maker who works from a strictly utilitarian position and the one who works from a deonologist will consider duties in relation to moral principles and "do what is right." Each position has limitations that need to be recognized by decision makers.

C.   PREVENTIVE ETHICS

This structure can be used for consideration of ethical dilemmas in interdisciplinary and intradisciplinary learning settings. However, the dimension of available time restricts discussions of ethical dilemmas. Nurses and students need time in which to do reflective thinking of this kind.

It seems critical that nurses have planned opportunities, in an unharrassed setting to structure specific and recurrent ethical dilemmas so that they can go beyond the agonizing conflict of wondering what to do or hoping that particular events do not happen when they are "on."

The format of "ethical rounds" can be used to reflect on and clarify the elements of decision making and ethical issues and dilemmas in hypothetical or actual situations. They can also offer nurses an opportunity to discuss how ethical dilemmas and issues differ for the nurse, vis-a-vis other health professionals, and the patient in bureaucratic structures. Further, they can be used to being medicine and nursing together to discuss and articulate the professional values and viewpoints each discipline brings to the situation.

One may take an additional step and ask, Are all ethical dilemmas that occur in nursing and health care inevitable? Is there such a thing as preventive ethics in nursing and health care? Such a concept could provide health workers with another way of considering ethical dilemmas.

For example, in nursing research involving human subjects, how many ethical dilemmas can be avoided through careful research design which would anticipate them? In practice, how many ethical dilemmas could be prevented through thoughtful assessment and careful listening to patients and families as they move through such difficult experiences as dying, living with a disability, or seeking painful information? Nurses are on this journey, too. To determine the anatomy of an ethical dilemma is to take the first step.

D. THE PRACTICE

Ms. W, an 80-year-old widow, has been hospitalized with pneumonia. She has diabetes and progressive circulatory complications. She has been treating an ulcer on her left leg at home. She lives alone and has been very independent with minimal help from neighbors. While hospitalized for the pneumonia, she develops a diabetic gangrene of her left foot. Her physician has called a surgical consult. The surgeon decides that an above-the-knee amputation is necessary. Ms. W is adamantly against the amputation, saying that she wants to die "whole." A nurse overhears her conversation with the surgeon, and later Ms. W. tells the nurse, "I'm not signing anything, I don't want my leg cut off." The surgeon says that he will have Ms. W's nephew sign for the amputation if Ms. W won't sign herself. He says that Ms. W is just "an obstinate old woman who doesn't know what's best for her." Ms. W's only other relative is a brother who has been in a state mental hospital for years. When the nurse expresses concern, the head nurse tells her that this is an issue between the patient and the surgeon and that she should not interfere.

[This case] presents an ethical dilemma for the nurse. She feels that she should do something as an advocate for the patient's right to self-determination, but the head nurse has made it clear that she should not interfere. As far as the staff nurse knows, the surgeon sees no alternative to the amputation, which he says is in the patient's best interest. The nurse is in conflict vis-á-vis the patient, the surgeon, and the head nurse.

Data Base

To begin to dissect this dilemma, the nurse can organize the information into a framework for decision making, as shown in Figure 10.2. She

Data Base	
Who are the actors involved? What are their histories and involvement in the situation?	**Patient**—advised by the surgeon that she must have an amputation to treat diabetic gangrene, has refused and stated she wants to die "whole"; **Hospital staff** and **consulting surgeon**—interested in providing care to prolong the patient's life, little or no involvement with patient as a person, unlikely to have any future involvement with patient as a person; **Head nurse**—interested in running a smooth functioning unit; **Primary nurse**—no prior involvement with patient; **Nephew**—not emotionally close to patient prior to her hospitalization; **Family physician**—has cared for the patient for almost 10 years.
What is the proposed action?	To amputate Ms. W's leg—with or without her consent.
What is the setting or context of the proposed action?	The patient has gone from relative independence at home to dependence in the hosptial. Amputation of her leg may impede her ability to continue her prehospital independence. The patient is in an acute care setting so the staff's involvement with her and her family will probably be short-term and whatever happens is not likely to have long-term effects on them.
What is the intention or purpose of the proposed action?	To prolong Ms. W's life.
What other alternatives or choices are available? What are the probable outcomes of each alternative and combinations?	• Discuss the situation further with the patient and try to persuade her to sign the consent for amputation. *Outcome?* Patient might consent if she can explore options without pressure or she might see the nurse's action as more pressure and become more adamant in her refusal. • Discuss the situation further with the surgeon and bring up the Patient's Bill of Rights posted in the hospital admissions office. *Outcome?* Surgeon might recognize the patient's right to make the decision and discuss it further with the patient or he might announce he doesn't believe in the bill of rights and inform the nurse it has no legal weight anyway. • Try to get in touch with the nephew before the surgeon contacts him. *Outcome?* Nephew might tell the surgeon and the surgeon might accuse the nurse of trying to subvert the physician-patient relationship. • Inform Ms. W's family physician of Ms. W's feelings about the proposed amputation. *Outcome?* Physician might say there isn't anything he can do since the amputation is absolutely essential. • Take the head nurse's advice and do nothing. *Outcome?* Nurse might avoid the risks of taking action and get along better with everyone or she might be seen as nonassertive.
What are the probable implications or consequences of the proposed action?	If the surgery is done without Ms. W's consent, she may retaliate aggressively by obtaining legal representation or passively by refusing to participate in the postoperative rehabilitation.

Figure 10.2 **Framework for Decision Making.**

Decision Theory Dimensions

/ho should decide? hysician, nurse, pa- ent, family commit- e? Why? For hom is the decision ade? Self or other?	• The patient should decide what happens to her own body. • The physician should decide for the patient, since he is doing what is in her best interests, and he has the technical expertise. • If the patient has been declared incompetent by some stated criterion, a guardian *ad litem* appointed by the court should decide for the patient, since the patient is unable to decide for herself.
'hat criteria should e used in deciding ho makes the deci- on? Social, legal, ychological, physio- gical, economic?	The nurse might: • Consider only Ms. W's physiological or medical status and choose to do nothing because she is convinced that only the physi- cian can assess the medical indication for the amputation. • Consider Ms. W's legal right, in the absence of an emergency or declaration of incompetency, to consent and help her get a lawyer. • Assess Ms. W's psychological reaction to amputation without her consent and try to delay the surgery until the patient agrees.
› what degree must ient *freely* consent?	What is the impact of consent obtained through coercion by the nephew or physician versus consent without coercion?
'hat, if any, moral inciples are en- nced or negated by proposed action?	• Abiding by the patient's refusal enhances the patient's right to self-determination; overriding it negates the right. • Obtaining the patient's consent enhances the principle of benefi- cence or nonmaleficence, as well as truthfulness.

Ethical Theories and Positions

Theory	Consideration	Decision-Making Logic
eontological hics/Formalist hics	The principles involved in the action: objective is to act "correctly" ac- cording to a moral princi- ple regardless of the consequences	There are moral principles that apply regard- less of the consequences. If the nurse does nothing, she "allows" an action which is harm- ful to Ms. W in that her dignity as an individ- ual will be violated and her body invaded with- out her consent. To do nothing conflicts with a principle of respect for the individual and her autonomy to make decisions about her own life and body. The nurse, coming from this ethi- cal position, *must do something*.
ilitarianism	The consequence of ac- tion on all involved now and in future: an action per se is neither right nor wrong, it becomes right when it produces the greatest happiness or the least harm for the greatest number.	To decide on an action, the consequences of each alternative must be considered and the one that provides the greatest happiness or the least harm for the greatest number selected. If the nurse does nothing, the physician, nephew, and head nurse will be "happy" because the patient's best interests, in their view, will have been served.
oism	Consequences of action on decision maker: ob- jective is to act so as to achieve the greatest hap- piness or least harm for self.	To decide on an action, the consequences of each alternative must be weighed in terms of the greatest good or least harm to the decision maker. If the nurse views herself as a patient advocate and does nothing, she risks psycho- logical harm. If nursing is a job, she will take the head nurse's advice and do nothing.

needs to gather as much data as she can about the situation, considering the questions in light of the people involved and the possible alternatives for action as well as their probable consequences. These do not exhaust all the possibilities, but the nurse should consider the following options: She can discuss the situation further with the patient, with the nephew, or with Ms. W's family physician, or she can take the head nurse's advice and do nothing. For each of the alternatives and combinations of alternatives, she must next consider the probable outcomes for all involved.

Decision theory dimensions

In addition to gathering the data, the nurse also needs to consider who should make the decision. Not everyone involved agrees that the patient should decide what happens to her own body. The patient claims that she should decide, while the physician claims that the decision is his, since he is doing what is in the patient's best interests, and he has the technical expertise.

A footnote, here, is that technical expertise cannot be generalized to the moral or ethical dimensions of a situation. In the hospital setting, the physician is in a position of power and authority; however, it cannot automatically be concluded that the physician or any other health professional is the best person to decide what is in the patient's best interest.

Even the courts have equivocated in situations involving the issue of rejecting treatment. A court might be asked to appoint a guardian *ad litem* for a decision about the proposed amputation *if* Ms. W had previously been declared "incompetent" by some stated criteria. It is very difficult to morally or legally justify the nephew or the physician making this decision for her.

Next, the nurse needs to reflect on *what* criteria should be used in choosing an alternative for action. For example, she might consider only Ms. W's physiological or medical status and choose to do nothing because she is convinced that only the physician can assess the medical indication for the amputation.

In terms of nursing's emphasis on the whole patient and the proclaimed role of the nurse or patient advocate, the nurse should also take into account the psychological, social, and spiritual dimensions of what the amputation means to Ms. W on a short- and long-term basis. In addition, she might take into consideration the economics of the situation and project the possible financial implications if Ms. W does or does not have the amputation. For example, what kinds of support systems might Ms. W need if she has the amputation and how will they be financed? The nurse might also think about the ordinary versus extraordinary-means distinction. Although this may appear to be important, it is often not very helpful in actually making decisions. What is ordinary in a large teaching hospital may be extraordinary in a small hospital. Identical treatment, such as giving antibiotics, may be ordinary in one situation and extraordinary in another.

If Ms. W did sign the consent form, the nurse might be concerned as to whether the decision was coerced by the nephew or the physician or freely made by the patient. This is not always an easy determination, but if the patient expresses doubts after signing the consent, the possibility of coercion and its implications need to be considered.

Additionally, the nurse would consider whether the possible alternatives enhanced or negated such principles as the patient's right to self-determination and the principle of beneficence or nonmaleficence. The latter principle says that one should not inflict harm or evil and that one ought to prevent harm, particularly intentional harm, or the risk of harm. This principle applies to patients and also requires that such agents as the physician and nurse are thoughtful about their actions and consider them in the light of professional standards. The nurse would judge which alternative best serves Ms. W. taking into consideration the standards of nursing practice.

Ethical Position

In considering various approaches, the nurse can look at the alternatives from different ethical theories or positions.

From a strictly utilitarian point of view, one would consider the possible consequences of each alternative and decide which alternative would provide the greatest amount of happiness for all concerned. For example, if she decides to do nothing, the physician, the nephew, and the head nurse presumably will be "happy" because the best interests of the patient, according to their assessment, have been served. Indeed, in some situations in which the physician has overruled the patient, the patient has been grateful later. One may not find this approach acceptable for a variety of reasons, including the lack of respect for the individual's autonomy. However, a strictly utilitarian approach might justify an alternative not justifiable under another ethical approach.

The strict deonotologist would say that there are moral principles that apply, regardless of the consequences. In Ms. W's situation, if the nurse firmly believes in a principle of respect for the individual's right to autonomously make decisions about his own life and body, the option of doing nothing to prevent others from forcing a decision on Ms. W. would not be justified. Also, in this context, doing nothing negates the principle of nonmaleficence by "allowing" an action that is harmful to the patient in the sense that her dignity as an individual will be violated and her body invaded without her expressed consent. For this nurse, a decision to do nothing would conflict with her moral principles. If, on the other hand, this nurse accepts the physician's option that the patient will die without the amputation and she believes in the value of maintaining life over individual autonomy, she may decide to participate in forcing Ms. W. to have the leg amputated.

Further, one can look at each alternative in light of whether or not it meets the tests of universality, generality, and publicity. Is the patient being treated as an end as well as a means? or is the patient being used to satisfy a health professional's ego needs? Is the nurse willing to let all involved know what she is doing? Is she willing to universalize this choice to others in similar circumstances?

Using a rights approach, the nurse might claim that she has the right and responsibility to be an advocate for the patient's point of view. She would choose an alternative that creates a situation in which the patient's feelings are made known and respected by all. The patient's right to reject treatment would be respected with the caveat that her decision was made after careful deliberation.

E.   DIMENSIONS OF TIME AND VALUES

Identifying the values of all involved in the situation is another dimension of clarifying a dilemma. If this nurse values obedience to those above her in the bureaucracy, she will follow the advice of her superior in the nursing hierarchy, the head nurse, and do nothing. If the nurse values self-determination for herself as a professional person and for clients as an overriding value, she will be unable to justify doing nothing, she will choose an alternative expressive of this value The nurse, the patient, and other health workers may hold different values about the nurse's role, about living with a mutilated body, or about any other factors involved.

The time element in Ms. W's situation is not as critical as in such situations as a cardiac arrest, in which the decision to resuscitate or not to resuscitate must be made in a very limited period of time. The nurse could use this framework for analyzing the dilemma either alone or with a colleague to reflect on Ms. W's situation and available options. She might even use it for a discussion with Ms. W's physician.

How and when a nurse looks at the anatomy of an ethical dilemma is related to time and values. Because of time, dilemmas must sometimes be resolved now and dissected later. But whether the nurse in Ms. W's situation analyzes the dilemma before or after acting may be more closely related to her values. Nurses hold different values in relation to using a deliberative and reflective thinking process *prior* to making decisions versus justifying decisions and actions *after* the fact. Thoughtful and careful reflection *before* taking action could fulfill one aspect of the principle of non-maleficence, that is, preventing intentional harm.

ENDNOTES

1. William K. Frankena, Ethics, 2nd ed.; Englewood Cliffs: Prentice-Hall, 1973, pp. 30–31.
2. John Rawls, Theory of Justice; Cambridge: Harvard, 1971, pp. 131–135.

CHAPTER 11

A BIOETHICAL DECISION MODEL

Joyce E. Thompson and Henry O. Thompson

In every encounter with clients or patients, professional colleagues and friends, there is a need to reason critically, to make ethical decisions. Professional nursing practice requires sound decision making at all levels of interaction and in all areas of nursing practice. To be professional is to be ethical. We have an ethical mandate to make good decisions. Just how we carry out that ethical mandate is the subject of this paper.

We have all learned *how* to make decisions as we grew up. Our nursing role requires that we also make decisions with and, sometimes for others. Is there any difference in the way we approach decision making as health care professionals [HCP] compared to personal decisions? Are we held to a higher standard of critical, moral reasoning because we are caring for others than when we care for ourselves? Ideally the response should be, "No" to both queries, but let us explore the concept of decision making.

FACTORS THAT FACILITATE GOOD DECISION MAKING

One approach to examining how people make decisions is to describe factors that facilitate good decisions and those that hinder or constrain one's decision making. The factors that promote good decision making include (1) time, (2) information gathering, (3) alternatives available, (4) knowledge of risks, costs, and benefits, (5) short and long term effects of a given choice or action, and (6) knowledge of one's own values and priorities and how these influence one's choices. Inherent in this process of good decision making is a commitment to analyze or critically think about the needed decision before taking action or making a choice. If time is limited or motivation to reason critically lacking, bad

Reprinted with permission from Thompson and Thompson, *Bioethical Decision Making for Nurses,* Appleton-Century-Crofts, E. Norwalk, Conn., 1985.

decisions may result. If those decisions affect only ourselves, we might be resigned to accept the consequences of a bad outcome. However, HCP are expected to avoid poor decisions and bad outcomes whenever possible. The consequences of these decisions affect others—especially patients we are taking care of. Therefore, some might respond to our earlier question that HCP are indeed held to a higher standard of decision making—at minimum, always using a critical reasoning process even when time is limited.

The concept of moral reasoning is one way of defining the elements of critical thinking. These elements include (1) analysis—examining the situation, sorting the ethical issues, and considering possible actions; (2) weighing—assessing the strengths and weaknesses of each proposed alternative, (3) justifying—identifying the reasons supporting the proposed action and those supporting not choosing other actions, (4) choosing—willing to and actually taking action or making a choice, including responsibility for outcomes, and (5) evaluating—looking at the results; were they expected or is another decision needed.

Many will quickly recognize the elements of the problem-solving process in both these approaches to good/ethical decision making. Thus moral reasoning and ethical decision making are not new concepts to nurses, though not often described in the terms used here.

FACTORS THAT HINDER OR CONSTRAIN GOOD DECISION MAKING

Factors that can negatively influence or constrain decision making include (1) personal values, (2) level of moral development, (3) limited understanding of ethical theory and principles, (4) lack of time, (5) lack of experience/expertise/maturity, (6) law, (7) conflicting loyalties and obligations, (8) cultural mores, (9) lack of decision-making capacity, and (10) lack of commitment to responsible choices and actions. Responsible HCP are aware that many of these factors are present in daily work. Their goal is to recognize them and try to minimize their negative effects on good decision making. Ignorance of such factors, however, does allow for bad decision making and hence, unethical practice.

A BIOETHICAL DECISION MODEL

Recognizing that critical inquiry and moral reasoning are essential elements of good decision making in health and illness care practice, the authors developed a decision model to guide professionals through the decision process. This model incorporates decision theory, moral analysis, applied ethical theory as well as both the factors that support and those that hinder or constrain good decision making in clinical practice.

The model that follows has been revised several times since its first trials in 1975 in keeping with new knowledge as well as longterm experiential use by and feedback from clinicians and educators. This model represents a *process* of decision making, not a prescription for the "right" choice. We cannot guarantee that if you follow each of the steps of the decision model, you will have a clear understanding of what path of action or choice to make when you finish. We do not guarantee that such a choice will be the ethical one. But we can assure you that your efforts will bring you closer to good decision making.

The final choice in any clinical situation will depend on one's knowledge of ethics, available alternatives and the potential outcomes of alternatives, legal, value and loyalty constraints as well as the clinician's and client's commitment to truthtelling and responsible participation in the decision process. Trust, mutual respect, and information sharing are inherent in the effective use of this or any other ethical decision model. These are also important elements of HCP/client relationships within which good decisions can be made. Professional nursing requires ethical decision making, and we offer the following as one model or process for nurses committed to critical thinking and ethical nursing practice.

GUIDELINES FOR IDENTIFYING AND ANALYZING ETHICAL DIMENSIONS OF HEALTH CARE PRACTICE

J.E. THOMPSON AND H.O. THOMPSON*

[A bioethical decision model offering a 10-step process for identifying and analyzing ethical aspects of health and illness care situations.]

Step One: Review the situation as presented to determine:
        a. health problems
        b. decision(s) needed
        c. key individuals

Step Two: Gather additional information to:
        a. clarify situation

---

*These guidelines are adapted from Thompson, J.E. and Thompson, H.O. *Bioethical Decision Making for Nurses*. Norwalk: Appleton-Century-Crofts, 1985, p. 99, with editorial changes in Fall 1988. Reprinted with permission.

           b. understand what information is missing

           c. understand legal constraints, if any

Step Three: Identify the ethical issues or concerns in the situation:

           a. explore historical roots of each

           b. explore current philosophical/religious bases

           c. explore current societal views on each issue

Step Four: Identify personal values and professional moral positions on issues/concerns identified in Step Three, including:

           a. review of personal constraints raised by the issues

           b. review of professional code for guidance

           c. identification of conflicting loyalties/obligations

Step Five: Identify moral positions of key individuals involved:

           a. through discussion of same

           b. by reviewing advance directives if available

Step Six: Identify value conflicts, if any and:

           a. attempt to understand bases for conflict

           b. explore means for possible resolution

Step Seven: Determine who is best able to make the needed decision(s):

           a. identify role of patient/client

           b. identify role of patient family/significant others

           c. identify role of health professional(s)

           d. identify role of specialized consultants such as clergy, social worker, lawyer

Step Eight: Identify the range of possible actions:

           a. describe anticipated outcome for each action

           b. include moral justification for each action

           c. decide which actions fit criteria for decision making in this situation

           d. determine how closely suggested actions conform to one's professional code of ethics

Step Nine: Decide on a course of action and carry it out:

           a. know reasons for choice of action

           b. explain reasons to others

           c. establish time frame for review of outcomes

Step Ten: Evaluate the results of decision/action:

           a. did expected outcomes occur?

           b. is new decision needed?

           c. was decision process complete?

           d. is further information needed? (begin again)

BIBLIOGRAPHY

These guidelines were originally based on the following:

Rebecca Bergman, "Ethics—Concepts and practice," *International Nursing Review* 20, No. 5 (1973), 140–141, 152.

M.A. Murphy, and J. Murphy, "Making ethical decisions—Systematically," *Nursing* 6, No. 6 (May 1976), OG 13–14.

David Belgum, *When Its Your Turn to Decide*. Minneapolis: Augsburg, 1978, 44f.

CHAPTER 12

MORAL DEVELOPMENT AND CLINICAL DECISION MAKING

Marsha D. Fowler and Kathleen A. Mahon

[Ethical analysis sometimes focuses on issues such as abortion. Another approach is to consider the moral agent. Kohlberg's concept of moral development offers a way of understanding why people do what they do, and in turn suggests an analysis of clinical decision making. Nursing education can provide a context for moral development.]

The choice of nursing interventions is usually thought to be based upon the nurse's scientific or theoretical knowledge, previous clinical experience, and personal capabilities, as well as the patient situation. Increasingly, however, there is greater cognizance of the role of "personal" variables in clinical decision making in nursing. These variables include personal values and beliefs, ethics, and, in particular, the stage of moral development of the nurse. The field of philosophical ethics includes any consideration of values, facts, and beliefs, while moral development considers the psychological processes of moral decision making. It is this process of resolving moral dilemmas that has great implications for nursing practice and nursing education.

Building upon the work of Jean Piaget, Lawrence Kohlberg has theorized that there are three levels, each in two stages, of moral development of the individual. While still in the process of verification and documentation, Kohlberg's levels of moral development may serve as a useful tool for nursing instructors who must assist their students in solving clinical moral dilemmas. It is the purpose of this paper to examine the clinical usefulness of Kohlberg's theory in facilitating instructor understanding and assessment of students' moral decision-making processes, and in establishing a moral milieu that will facilitate growth in that process.

From *Nursing Clinics of North America*, 14, no. 1, March 1979, 3–12. Reprinted with permission of W. B. Saunders Company.

A. KOHLBERG'S THEORY OF MORAL DEVELOPMENT

Kohlberg divides moral development into three levels: preconventional, conventional, and postconventional. Each of these levels is further subdivided into two numbered stages, one stage being more organized than the other and more advanced in determining what is "right" or "good". Even though progression through the stages may occur over varying lengths of time, they are seen to be invariably sequential.(1) Research supports the thinking that "once a person has adopted a higher stage of (moral) reasoning, he may still offer lower stage responses to questions, but he generally accepts only higher reasons as determinative and will not lose higher orientation once he has developed.(2)

Preconventional Level of Moral Development

The preconventional level, so called because individuals within its two stages do not consciously attend to society's norms when responding to problems, is represented by both stage one and stage two. Stage one individuals have a punishment-and-obedience orientation. Because this is something of a comfort-oriented stage, this person responds to the threat of punishment, especially physical or that determined by another's authority, with obedience. "Right" and "wrong" are determined by what the person wants versus the envisioned consequence of the action in terms of reward or punishment. "Right" or "good" is dependent upon another's ability to force. The person in this stage and succeeding stages cannot understand the moral reasoning of others who are more than one stage above his own.(3) The following is an example of a stage one response.

Nurse A, with the help of one nursing assistant, is assigned to care for 21 seriously ill medical patients on a medical unit. When faced with the choice to stay and give minimal care or to refuse to work under such conditions, she decided to remain. Her stated reason for remaining was, "If I leave they will fire me, and I'll get a bad reference."

Stage two persons are pragmatically opportunistic. The orientation in this stage is toward the more concrete ideas of direct and immediate reciprocation or retaliation, without the intrusion of more abstract concepts such as duty, honor, or justice. Stage two persons establish a tit-for-tat type of relationship that may involve bargaining but is mostly directed at personal ascendency or gain. In both stage one and stage two, the fear of physical consequences and of the power exerted by those in authority determines the nature of right and wrong. While this is true of both stages, in level two the person shows a willingness to cooperate or bargain with others while being overtly or covertly self-seeking. A stage two response may be seen in the following example.

Nurse B has among her patients a demanding elderly woman who constantly has her call light on. She has "Seconal h.s. repeat × 1" ordered. Having given one Seconal, Nurse B elects to give the second Seconal, which is equivocally necessary, because "she keeps leaning on the light and I'm tired of answering her little complaints. Besides, a second one was ordered p.r.n."

Conventional Level of Moral Development

Stage three marks the conventional level, wherein the individual conforms to societal expectations or demands and seeks to maintain the social status quo. The third stage is classically typified by those who acquiesce to peer and social pressures to gain the reward of social approval. This person attempts to meet stereotypical expectations of "good" behavior in both individual and group situations. Important others are those with whom the individual has personal dealings, rather than unknowns. For the first time, the question of motivation enters in. "Good" and "bad" now become at least partly based upon the person's intent; failure to meet the stereotypical standard may be adjudged as "unfortunate," but no less "good" in the presence of sincere intention. In this stage, the consequences of pain or punishment may be endured willingly in an attempt to fulfill the expectations of the stereotype. Level three responses are typified by this example.

Head Nurse C is responsible for orienting recent graduate, Nurse D. She has informed Nurse D that patient Smith's doctor prefers a particular brand of irrigating bag and tubing. Nurse D, while hanging the proper solution, inadvertently chooses the standard bag and tubing, since the brand of bag was not specified in the orders. On rounds, Head Nurse C says to the doctor, "I explained to her that you like the other bags, but I accept full responsibility for her mistake. I'll take care of this for you right away and talk with Nurse D so that she'll get it straight next time. New graduates are all alike. They ignore the doctor's preferences."

Stage four is dominated by a law-and-order mentality and contains many of the same elements—conformity and maintenance of status quo—as stage three. The difference between the stages lies in the object of conformity. Stage three involves conformity to persons, whereas stage four is dominated by conformity to rules, whether civil (legal) or moral. This also includes conformity to rules established by organizations or institutions with which the person is affiliated. "Wrong" action is defined as violation of these rules, regardless of the consequences and, more important, irrespective of the reasonableness of content of that rule. Moral decisions are unyielding, and social order is seen as being good in and of itself. In stage four, the fear of loss or absence of social approval is replaced by "official" punishment in the forms of incarceration, citation, and exclusion. In the preconventional and conventional levels, responses are determined by external factors. An example of stage four moral development follows.

The doctor has ordered that the patient not be told about drug side effects "because the family doesn't want to discuss it." Yet the family has repeatedly asked Nurse E to talk with them about the patient's iatrogenic condition and therapy. Despite the need that the family demonstrates, Nurse E refuses to discuss the patient's drugs "because the doctor ordered us not to."

Postconventional Level of Moral Development

The postconventional level of development involves more internal and autonomous modes of thinking than the other stages. The movement from stage one to stage six demonstrates a conceptual movement, the higher stages being considerably more advanced cognitively.(4) According to Kohlberg, "There is a clear effort to define moral values and principles which have validity and application apart from the authority of the groups or persons holding these principles, and apart form the individual's own identification with these groups."(5) Not until a person enters stage five does he recognize that there exist mutually exclusive, competing rights and values within moral conflicts. This is the "social contract" stage in which the individual views the law as a binding code of behavior with content that can be changed by the will of the majority when necessary for utilitarian, rational, or updating purposes. It is in this stage that such shared concepts as duty, welfare of the majority, basic human rights, democracy, and constitutionality come into effect. Beyond the guidelines of democratically chosen rules, "right" is personally determined by conscience.(6)

Stage five moral development is seen the following example.

Nurse F is caught in a situation in which the primary physician has deceived the family regarding the patient's prognosis. The family is now asking Nurse F to verify the physician's remarks. Dual "loyalties" are at conflict in this nurse—loyalty to the physician and loyalty to the patient.

Hospital guidelines indicate that she should support the physician's "judgement" in this situation, but the patient's family's right to the truth is a competing claim. Nurse F opted to give an evasive answer that supported the physician's general abilities. She later stated to the other staff members, "I'll talk with Dr. G and see if we can work this out. The family needs and has a right to know about the patient's status. I don't think it's right to string them along."

Here, the nurse felt that the institution's claim (and the physician's) was stronger but, feeling that deception was wrong, decided to work to change the physician's mind.

Stage six goes beyond stage five in that it entails the application of universal ethical principles that are self-chosen, comprehensive, consistent, logical, and universal. Because of the universality of these principles, the person's life has a great deal of consistency or congruence not found in other stages. These principles generally emanate from the person's philosophy of life, which will demonstrate characteristics of breadth, depth, comprehensiveness, and coherence. In this stage, duty exists within the realm of these principles rather than being defined by contractual or legalistic agreement. Stage six involves a higher degree of abstraction than previous stages, and in situations of conflict, these abstract principles supersede the demands of law. The individual in stage six commits himself to his principles, which are at least somewhat heuristic or open to alteration; failure in application of these principles is seen to reflect upon the person rather than upon the adequacy of the principle.

Stage six of moral reasoning is displayed in the following example:

Nurse researcher H has been conducting a research project for which it has been difficult to locate suitable subjects. Patient I is an ideal subject, but because he is comatose he cannot give informed consent. The research project will neither harm nor hurt the patient and will not involve any cost to him. The patient's wife and physicians have given permission to use this patient. Nurse H, having to decide whether or not to involve the patient, opts not to, feeling that if she did it "would violate the patient's dignity by using him as an instrument rather than an end in and of himself."

These, then are Kohlberg's six stages of moral development in overview.(7) It must again be pointed out that in any given situation there may be agreement regarding what should be done, but the underlying rationale will differ markedly. It is the moral reasoning of the person rather than the actual decision made that is of concern in examining an individual's moral development.

B. STAGE ANALYSIS

Because nursing is a clinical profession, formal nursing education generally occurs both in group and in individual settings. Being concerned primarily with group learning experiences, this article cannot give more than passing attention to an analysis of this individual's stage of moral development. Various tools have been designed to test individually for a person's stage of development; even so, it can be a difficult task. Often subtle differences between the stages, differences in interpersonal communication, and multistage responses from one individual combine to complicate stage assessment. To some extent, identification of a specific stage of development may not be critically necessary. A general understanding of the stages will at least permit the instructor to determine the level rather than the stage. Within the context of plenary lectures, seminars, or discussions, it is generally more useful for the instructor to attempt to ascertain the general development level of the group in order to deal with responses collectively.(8) Of course, some persons will not be in concert with the majority of the group; ideally these students would be attended to on a more individual basis.

At this juncture, a word should be said about the dangers of stage analysis, which include inaccurate analysis and labeling. Variations in personal communication style and ability to articulate reasoning may cause a student's statements to resemble those characteristic of a particular stage. The student's moral reasoning may in actuality represent a different stage. Labeling, whether accurate or not, has several attendant perils. Bolt and Sullivan write of self-fulfilling prophecies that arise from differential treatment as a result of labeling. They further speak of "creating expectancy advantages and disadvantages" when labels are employed.(9) The instructor runs the risk of "freezing" a student in a particular stage or eliciting a Hawthorne effect if she regards students by label (i.e. skewing results to meet a researcher's expectations).

In determining the general level of moral development of the group, one can gather information that will assist in establishing a moral milieu designed to facilitate growth. Research into the effects of classroom moral education upon the moral development of children and adolescents has shown that such exposure tends to move students toward a higher level of thinking.(10) Kohlberg has found that a "just community" program conducted in a women's prison "led to an upward change in moral reasoning as well as to later changes in life-style and behavior."(11) Research further indicates that "transition from one stage to another is most likely to occur when a person is: (1) challenged with moral problems for which his stage of thinking provides no easy answers, and (2) presented with responses a stage higher than his own."(12)

C. MORAL DEVELOPMENT AND NURSING EDUCATION

In one study, two groups of 10 nursing students were studied relative to individual changes in stage of moral development. The control group was studied during a five-week pediatrics rotation immediately following an obstetrics rotation. The experimental group was studied during the obstetrics rotation, having just completed pediatrics. Students had been randomly assigned to groups at the beginning of the school year. The independent variable was exposure of the experimental group to specific, planned moral content in a very brief "nursing rounds" format. Owing to the nature of the content of both courses, all students were equally exposed to some ethical content in lectures. Lecture topics which were covered included: congenital deformities and handicaps, abortion, birth control, sterilization, institutionalization of the mentally handicapped, child abuse, and others.

Using the Defining Issue Test, students were pre- and post-tested to measure moral judgment development. The Defining Issue Test (DIT) is an objective test that presents stimulated moral dilemmas and asks the student to rank and rate 12 issues (questions) according to their relative importance with respect to the story. Subjects are also asked to mark "yes," "no," or "can't decide" for how they think characters in the story should respond.

The subjects are scored on a "P-score per cent." or P%, which "is interpreted as the relative importance a subject gives to principal moral considerations in making a decision about moral dilemmas." It is a sum per cent of weighted ranks given to stages 5 and 6.

A statistically significant difference was found between the control and experimental groups. The increase in level of moral judgment development of the experimental group was found to be significantly greater (P = .05) than that of the control group.

A second significant finding of the study relates to the scores of the students tested. Rest has found that scores average in the 40's for college underclassmen, in the 50's for upperclassmen, in the 60's for graduate students, and in the 70's for academic specialists in the moral, social, and political science disciplines. For both groups, the average scores of the nursing students were higher on post-test than for college students at an equivalent level. This may reflect the clinical nature of a nursing course of study, including its inherent repeated exposure to moral dilemmas in which the student must participate.

An additional observation made during the study related to the increase in frequency of expressions of moral outrage among the students in the experimental group. Subsequent to the study, those students in the experimental group correctly identified moral dilemmas in the clinical setting more frequently. These students further demonstrated greater ability to differentiate moral dilemmas from legal, social, and other issues. The identification of ethical questions and the expression of moral outrage occurred even when the student stated that he would not have changed his course of action in a given situation. It is the feeling of these researchers that these changes as well as the upward changes in moral judgment warrant continued investigation and increased attention to establishing a milieu in which moral development may progress.

D.   ESTABLISHING A MORAL MILIEU

The goal of establishing a moral milieu is to facilitate growth in moral development. Objectives that would need to be met along the way include instructor recognition of moral decisions as such, acquisition of understanding of the stages of moral reasoning, identification of those stages when they were expressed, and in provision of elements of student experience previously missed.(14) Student experience is supplemented with planned content, often utilizing a case study method.

Several studies have linked moral judgment made on objective tests to moral action. It is therefore not unrealistic to assume this approach in a classroom setting. Blatt and Kohlberg stress two major principles in moral education: "the arousal of genuine moral conflict, uncertainty, and disagreement about genuinely problematic situations" and "the presentation of modes of thought one stage above the child's own." While it has been suggested that the critical period for intervention in moral development is the preadolescent period, later intervention is not without effect. Blatt and Kohlberg indicate that intervention between ages 10 and 14, when the child is typically moving from the preconventional to the conventional level, can prevent stabilization at the preconventional level by those who might be so disposed.(15)

Several conditions have been identified as being involved in creating a moral milieu:(16)

1. Establish fairness in rules and group process in the program. Conflicts should be treated as issues in justice and fairness.

2. Create a climate of trust and openness in sharing. An explicit degree of confidentiality should exist, particularly if cases are real rather than contrived.
3. Focus on moving the group as a group in its moral development.
4. Stimulate individual moral decisions by serving as facilitator rather than as the final authority.
5. Share the principles and theory of moral development with the students. This will assist in creating a sense of common goals, responsibilities, and authority.

These principles have been adapted from work with prisoners to an educational setting. In addition to the abovementioned principles, several teaching methods and strategies have been found to be particularly useful in classroom settings with nursing students.(17) Ethics rounds, which entails the classroom presentation of various ethical concepts as well as moral development materials, has proven to be particularly helpful when used in a case study method of presentation. Actual cases are used (some in which the students are currently involved) to facilitate personal identification with the material as well as clinical relevance. When the student can be "hooked" into this sort of identification, role-playing usually becomes superfluous. Student-directed discussions, in which the student is responsible for bringing in his own case study, encourage an atmosphere of mutual participation and authority and encourage the student to identify moral dilemmas in his own practice. Logical analyses of situations should be encouraged, heightened cognitive conflict. Generally, when a case study discussion is undertaken all stages of moral reasoning (usually except stage one) may be in evidence. When this occurs, everyone in the group is exposed to moral reasoning at least one level above his own.

E.   CONCLUSION

From a purely theoretical vantage point, moral development theory is concerned with reasons and rationale for actions or decisions, rather than the decisions themselves. However, within the context of applied theory in the clinical setting, those decisions that affect patient or staff well-being must of necessity be taken into consideration. That is, in the clinical setting, both the process and the content become important—the former for theoretical considerations, and the latter for health considerations.

Current theories of moral development are still in the stages of testing and validation. Kohlberg's theory provides a useful tool in the clinical education of nursing students. It is equally applicable to nurses in practice. Unfortunately, knowledge of Kohlberg's theory will not make moral decisions themselves any easier; hard decisions will always have to be made. It will, however, enable the clinical instructor to analyze various responses to moral dilemmas. This will allow instructor response within the understanding of the student and, when set within a context of questioning and free expression, can hasten the growth in moral judgment of the persons involved. Ultimately, perhaps this will facilitate moral communication, bringing greater resources to bear upon those "hard cases" that are daily encountered in nursing practice.

ENDNOTES

1. Lawrence Kohlberg, "The child as moral philosopher," Psychology Today 2 (Sep 68), 25–30.

2. Robert Hall and John Davis, Moral Education in Theory and Practice; Buffalo, NY: Prometheus Books, 1975.

3. Ronald Duska and Mariellen Whelen, Moral Development. A Guide to Piaget and Kohlberg; NY: Paulist Press, 1975.

4. Kohlberg, "Moral Stages and Moralization," pp.31–53 in Moral Development and Behavior ed. Thomas Likona; NY: Holt, Rinehart and Winston, 1976.

5. Kohlberg, "From Is to Ought," in Cognitive Development and Epistemology ed. T. Mischel; NY: Academic Press, 1971.

6. Kohlberg, Kelsey Kauffman, Peter Scharf, and Joseph Hickey, "The just community approach to corrections: A theory," Journal of Moral Education [JME] 4, No. 3 (June 75), 243–260.

7. More recently, Kohlberg has theorized that there is a transitional phase 4 ½ and a stage 7 (religion). A reevaluation showed that there is a lack of data for stage 6 but he currently keeps it as a theoretical stage.

8. Hall and Davis, op. cit.

9. Daniel J. Bolt and Edmund V. Sullivan, "Kohlberg's cognitive-developmental theory in educational settings: Some possible abuses," JME 6, No. 3 (May 77), 198–205.

10. Moshe Blatt and Kohlberg, "The effects of classroom moral discussion upon children's level of moral judgment," JME 4, No. 2 (Feb 75), 129–161.

11. Kohlberg, Moral Stages., op. cit.

12. Hall and Davis, op. cit.

13. Kathleen Mahon and Marsha Fowler, "Changes in moral judgment in junior nursing students." Unpublished research, 1978. James Rest, Manual for Defining Issues Test; Minneapolis: University of Minnesota, 1974. Id., Moral Development: Advances in Research and Theory; NY: Praeger, 1986.

14. Helen Weinreich, "Kohlberg and Piaget: Aspects of their relationship in the field of moral development," JME 4, No. 3 (June 75), 201–213.

15. Blatt and Kohlberg, Effects of classroom . . , op. cit.
16. Kohlberg, et al., Just Community . . , op. cit.
17. Mahon and Fowler, op. cit.

For additional study, see Kohlberg, Essays on Moral Development, Vol. 1 (1981). The Philosophy of Moral Development, and, 2 (1984). The Psychology of Moral Development; San Francisco: Harper & Row.

SECTION V
PROFESSIONAL RELATIONSHIPS

CHAPTER 13

NURSING RIGHTS

Claire M. Fagin

[The focus of nurses' rights has often been on the right not to do, e.g., Senator Church's amendment which protects such a right. "Now it is time to grasp the right to *do*." Nurses' rights are set in a context of women's rights and human rights. Rights have a corollary responsibility. It is not enough to get rights—nurses need to be alert to keeping their rights.]

The notion that nurses have rights has emerged strongly, and, if anything, is gaining momentum. Years ago, when I was a master's student in psychiatric nursing, my instructor, Hildegard Peplau, introduced us to the notion that nurses had a right to follow their beliefs in participating in patient's treatment. Specifically, we discussed the participation of nurses in electroshock therapy. It was incomprehensible to most of us that we could opt for nonparticipation with physicians in this or any other therapy when we were the employees of a hospital or other health agency. Nevertheless, some brave souls did act on their convictions with varying degrees of success. Within that context, nurses' rights could be defined as a refusal to participate in situations in conflict with their preparation, competencies, and beliefs. This is the right not to do rather than the right to do.

Recent statements or resolutions on rights in nursing practice have grown out of concerns of nurses regarding the abortion issue and their rights in this matter. Again, this involves a right not to do rather than a right to do. Many of the current resolutions regarding the rights of nurses are entitled, "Rights and Responsibilities of Nurses." Few rights are stated that do not have a concomitant responsibility, with the single exception of the refusal to participate. The statements of rights issues by the International Council of Nurses and various state nurses' organizations seem to confuse rights with responsibilities, with that single exception. Nurses' rights, as defined by our organizations, seem to me a kind of double talk on nurses' duties and responsibilities.

The resolution on nurses' rights issued by the Michigan State Nurses' Association has become the model in present usage throughout the United States. The listing of rights in resolution form are as follows:

RESOLVED, That the nurse practitioner has the responsibility to inform employers, present and prospective, of her educational preparation, experience, clinical competencies and those ethical beliefs which would affect her practice, and be it,

RESOLVED, That the nurse practitioner has the responsibility to alter, adjust to or withdraw from situations which are in conflict with her preparation, competencies and beliefs, and be it,

RESOLVED, That the employer shall provide the resources through which health services are made available to the recipient, and be it,

RESOLVED, That the nurse practitioner has the right and responsibility to collaborate with her/his employer to create an environment which promotes and assures the delivery of optimal health services, and be it further,

RESOLVED, That the nurse has the right to expect that her/his employer will respect her/his competencies, values and individual differences as they relate to her/his practice(1)

Only the last two statements deal with what I understand as "rights."

A.   RIGHTS VERSUS RESPONSIBILITY

As usually stated, so-called "rights of nurses" make me wonder whether my conception of rights is somewhat off the mark. However, the dictionary, thesaurus, and a handbook of synonyms validate my right to confusion since the actual definitions of rights and responsibilities do not support the blurring nurses' writings would suggest.

The word "right" is defined as a just claim to anything to which one is entitled such as power or privilege. A "right" is that which one may properly demand or claim as just, moral, or legal. A close synonym to right is prerogative.

The word "responsible" on the other hand, means to be accountable, to be answerable for something, to be liable, to be able to satisfy any reasonable claim involving important work or trust; a duty; a charge. It has also been defined as trustworthy, dependable, reliable, expected or obliged. The relationship between these two words, at least from the standpoint of their definitions, seems obscure but I do believe there is an interrelationship. It seems to me that nurses' groups reach the relationship more rapidly than others but, in the process of reaching it too rapidly, tend to lose the focus on rights and increase the focus on responsibilities.

Why does anyone or any group have rights? Are rights given to us at birth? Do we obtain them by virtue of what we do or what we are? Are rights inherited? The answers to these questions would have to be a qualified "yes." It would be difficult, however, to say that everyone in our society is born with rights other than a culturally defined minimum of rights for shelter, food, and education. Clearly, society grants special rights to some individuals or groups in exchange for something society sees of value to it. Individuals endowed with special rights by virtue of fortunate birth must also develop self-systems that enable them to perform those behaviors, which permit definition of the rights wanted and the methods of obtaining them.

It is clear that nursing history has militated against nursing's awareness and use of rights. Originally, nursing was identified as a religious vocation. This connotation of "service" and "calling" continued in secular nursing and combined with the role of women in society to create an almost impossible barrier of socialization which inhibited a striving for personal or professional rights. In recent years we have begun to give lip-service to the rights and prerogatives that we, as human beings and workers, possess. While we have finally allowed the words to pass our lips, our view of ourselves, from early patterning on, focuses on our responsibilities, duties, charges, and obligations to others.

Until recent years, persons in any of the helping fields, be it nursing, teaching or ministering, were not seen by society at large as having rights. It is exceedingly difficult for groups, products of their own society, to see themselves any differently from their cultural image. I believe this explains somewhat simplistically our confusion in this area as we attempt to delineate rights and then present papers filled with statements about responsibilities.

B.   HUMAN RIGHTS

Before defining nurses' rights let's focus first on human rights. Philosophically, the rights of a human being have to do with permitting humanness—feelings, inclinations, compassions, sympathies, intelligence, and thoughts. One's rights ought to involve the creation of situations to enhance humanness. Clearly, this would include the right to exercise one's abilities, the right to express oneself freely, the right to grow up as well as old, the right for fair compensation for one's work, and the right to obtain satisfaction in living. Furthermore, if to humanize is to help someone become kind, merciful, considerate, civilized, and refined, some reciprocal self-enhancement is required to meet this description in relation to others. Thus, rights of humans.

This approach is not original. Many groups are recognizing their lack of rights in the area of humanness and are making conscious efforts to obtain the human rights that they believe have been denied them. The women's rights movement is a case in point.

C.   WOMEN'S RIGHTS

The National Organization for Women, the largest feminist organization in the country, has a statement on rights which interestingly seems to close the circle between rights and responsibilities. According to NOW, the women's rights movements strives for equality and dignity for people through complete freedom of choice in pursuit of their life style and life goals, for access to leadership positions, equality of opportunity, equal pay, and self-determination. They strive to expose and change inequalities in the law, in discriminatory policy and practices, in prejudicial myths, and outdated attitudes. They consider equality a birthright and believe women have the right to be in the mainstream of American society, exercising privileges and responsibilities in a truly equal partnership with men. They are dedicated to the proposition that women are human beings, who, like all others in our society, have the right and the opportunity to develop their fullest human potential.(2)

In explaining why women have not been more active in securing human rights, NOW points out that women have been conditioned to accept limited and damaging self-concepts accompanied by low aspiration levels and lack of self-identity. One reason for their emphasis on consciousness-raising groups and publicity for their cause is that it is important to share the data regarding the extent of sex bias in everyday life and to help women, together, develop programs for change. In discussing why women ignore opportunities to improve their own lot they point out that women isolate themselves from one another, mistakenly assuming that their problems are personal rather than societal problems. They also point out that women fear losing male approval in our male dominated society. NOW believes that women can achieve equality only by accepting fully the responsibilities they share with all other persons in our society. In order to be part of the decision-making mainstream of American political, economic, and social life, women must create a new image of themselves by acting on their own and speaking out in behalf of their own equality, freedom, and human dignity. This is not to be interpreted as seeking special privileges nor as ". . . enmity toward men who are also victims of the current, half-equality between the sexes . . . but rather in the direction of an active, self-respecting partnership. . . . By so doing, women will develop confidence in their own ability to determine actively, in partnership with men, the conditions of their life, their choices, their future, and their society."(3)

In the statements of civil rights groups, consumer groups, and others seeking rights today, the similarities seem more important than the differences. The right to equal and full participation, the right to information and sharing of information, the right to personal growth, and the right to access to power, emerge in all of them. Except for some fortunate groups to whom society grants special rights by virtue of personal or professional inheritance, people seem to obtain rights by having an image of themselves as worthy of rights, through sharing positive information and publicity about themselves, through pressure, and through doing something for society which society values.

How then do nurses' rights differ from human rights or women's rights and where do our particular notions of responsibilities fit? It is interesting to substitute the word "nurses" for "women" in some of the rights statements of the women's movement. To paraphrase them, nurses will do most to create a new image of themselves by acting now and by speaking out in behalf of their own equality, freedom, and human dignity. This acting and speaking will not be in a plea for special privilege nor in enmity towards physicians and others who are also victims of the current inequality between the professionals, but rather in a direction of an active self-respecting partnership with them. In so doing, nurses will develop self-confidence in their own ability to determine actively, in partnership with other health professionals, the conditions of their life, choices, future, and society.

D. NURSES' RIGHTS

What then does the fact that all human beings have the right to self expression, to full participation, and to enactment of their special abilities, mean to us as nurses? What are our special rights as professionals? I would list the following rights:

1. The right to find dignity in self-expression and self-enhancement through the use of our special abilities and educational background.
2. The right to recognition for our contribution through the provision

of an environment for its practice, and proper, professional economic rewards.

3. The right to a work environment which will minimize physical and emotional stress and health risks.
4. The right to control what is professional practice within the limits of the law.
5. The right to set standards for excellence in nursing.
6. The right to participate in policy making affecting nursing.
7. The right to social and political action on behalf of nursing and health care.

I believe there is a direct relationship between human rights and these nurses' rights. Human refers to whatever is descriptive of man and the work "humane" is often used to describe an expectation about the nurse. If we consider the nurse's human rights in terms of professional rights, we could list the right to be heard, the right to participate freely and effectively, the right to satisfaction, and the right to question or doubt. It is when these rights are not fulfilled, that we feel we are not being treated as human beings.

Nurses have made one clear statement of rights—the refusal to participate. To me, the *not* do, of our rights expression is significant. It's all too close to the level of learning expressed in developmental tasks where children learn who they are by saying they *don't* wish to do. This is an early step in self-development and in the differentiation aspects of who one is. I hope we can move through this step very rapidly and delineate what we have the right *to* do as well as not to do.

As June Rothberg has identified, our legal rights to practice and to exercise our professional rights are described in nurse practice acts and in a wealth of common law and tradition.(4) In every state of this nation, nurses are legally responsible for their actions and inactions. A key differentiation between nurses and other legally sanctioned health professionals has to do with the public's direct access to service.

One could easily state that there is a strong relationship between such direct access and power, privilege, and rights among the health professions. Society appears to grant rights for valued service directly given rather than service delivered through an intermediary. Without this direct relationship it is difficult for the public to become aware of what a group has to offer. The public sees nursing as a sub-branch of medicine, ordered and controlled by physicians. If they have received good nursing care in a hospital, for example, they frequently believe that this is the result of physician's orders or some other control outside the realm of nursing practice and decision making.

The law in many instances tends to support this delusion, if indeed it always is a delusion. For example, in order for nurses to be paid by Medicare for their services to patients at home they must have physician's orders for any or all nursing services rendered. Although states may legalize and sanction nurses making judgments about what nursing services patients require, nurses have not been given the right to make this judgment practicable.

The New York State Nurse Practice Act, for example, states that nursing is diagnosing and treating human responses to actual or potential health problems, through such services as case finding, health teaching, health counseling, and initiation of health care. There is power and leverage within this definition. Yet few nurses have so far shown evidence of grasping this inherent power and using it effectively. Nurses, for the most part, play the role described earlier of all women—submissive, dependent, indirect, and frightened. Failure to act on behalf of our rights increases our guilt and low self-esteem and compounds our problems by discouraging the development of enabling behaviors to achieve rights. In seeking security, rather than satisfaction, we are, more often than not, unaware of our lack of achievements. Many of our constituents view their jobs as eight hours of drudgery leading, hopefully, to satisfactions in other areas of life separated from work. In this process we lose the benefits of years of education, our original motivation in becoming nurses, and the potential value of most of our awake lives.

Rather than face this misery openly and honestly we have found it much easier to focus on the responsibilities we ought to have and not have. We are more likely to blame others for the fact that we are not able to carry out the responsibilities we describe in our own nursing literature or in the resolutions quoted earlier. Unfortunately, in this blaming of others we contribute to the alienation of professionals from each other and towards an ever expanding gulf of hostility and non-communication. This is not living, no less professional practice. This highest order of responsibility in our priority system should be the responsibility of seeing, through unified action, that our rights are obtained. Leadership in our educational and work situations is required in order to revise the socialization process of nurses and others towards active participation and self-realization. Rigid bureaucratic settings do not encourage active participation. Nor, however, do educational settings which claim to have eliminated the trappings of bureaucracy but through covert and overt messages encourage adjustment and adaptation rather than growth and learning. It behooves us all to examine the conditions of our professional lives in order to ferret out those which inhibit self-enhancement and capitalize on aspects which will encourage our goal of advancing nurses' rights. The climate is now conducive to this goal, providing society sees itself as gaining something in return.

E.   HOW TO KEEP RIGHTS

Nurses' rights and nurses' responsibilities come together, I believe in the sense that frequently the carrying out of responsibilities on behalf of others will enhance our power base by increasing our support. This broadened power base helps us obtain and keep the rights nurses ought to have in health care systems. For example, new federal guidelines for nursing homes have been issued which even further relax the not-so-high requirements for nursing. No meaningful publicity accompanied this event, How many of the affected individuals and their relatives are aware that the federal government has reduced the standards for nursing in nursing homes? How many nurses are aware that this relaxation not only affects the elderly but has enormous implications for their own livelihoods? Using our rights to act politically would involve a wide range of activities calculated to affect law-making groups on behalf of direct professional interests as well as our responsibilities to the people we are serving. This kind of demand for rights, pertaining to patient care, done noisily and publicly, will help to obtain and keep the power and leverage suggested in the new definitions of nursing practice. We cannot claim what is rightfully ours unless we demonstrate some answerability for our actions. To be responsible and accountable for the delivery of nursing, we must have the authority to act and to do what is necessary to deliver this essential service. We must, through direct action, convince the public that we have a service of great value to deliver. Presently, the public's dissatisfaction with medical and hospital services harbors the threat that some long held rights of power groups may be taken away. It therefore becomes vital, in obtaining and keeping nurses' rights as professionals, to set the highest possible standards for delivering quality nursing care. Consumer validation of our view of quality nursing will clearly have an effect on our rights and legitimacy.

POSTSCRIPT

I believe nurses are demanding their rights more in the late 1980s than they were in the middle 70s. Their demands are now tied to matters of quality of care more than to personal need. But I do also believe nurses have not gone far enough.

If nurses were demanding rights appropriately, why would the average percentage of time spent with patients in hospitals be 25% instead of 75%? Why would nurses not be demanding 24 hour coverage of support services in every hospital? Why would nurses still be picking up responsibilities of other departments instead of demanding departmental accountability on behalf of patient care? Why would hospitals revolve around the physician staff and schedule patient activities, admissions, etc. for physician convenience rather than patient care priorities? Why would nurses' salaries be so compressed as with every other professional group?

Underlying any response to the questions I have raised is the sense of responsibility nurses have to the patient and to getting the job done in some way so that the patient's suffering is kept to an absolute minimum. Nurses' views of their own rights at the end of the 20th century continue to be confounded by a sense of responsibility to both the patient and the institution. The extreme nursing shortage of the early 1980s did not mobilize nurses to new demands for achieving rights. The nursing shortage of the late 1980s, much more severe, is creating widespread hysteria among hospital administrators and physicians.

Opportunities for collaborative action among nurses to solve plaguing problems of the profession abound. Many of these problems have to do with rights relating to professional nursing practice. Some progress is evident in salary and working conditions but the progress in no way matches the opportunities. Thus the conclusions of the original paper remain valid.

ENDNOTES

1. 1973 Convention issues: Proposed resolution = 1 on rights on responsibilities in nursing practice (News) Michigan Nurse Newsletter 46 (Sep 73), 26.

2. National Organization For Women, New York Chapter, What We're All About; NY: The Organization, 1973.

3. National Organization For Women, Statement of Purpose; Chicago: The Organization.

4. June S. Rothberg, Choosing to Use Your Professional Prerogatives. Paper presented at the Tennessee Nurses' Association Biennial Convention, held in Memphis, TN, 4 Oct 73.

CHAPTER 14

MODELS OF NURSE/PATIENT PHYSICIAN RELATIONS

Richard T. Hull

[Hull suggests three views of humanity—religious, individual, and community. Three models of patient-physician relationships follow—the priestly, the contractual, and the collegial. The corollary for the nurse's role in handmaiden for the first, a role largely rejected today. The third is the ideal but may not be realistic, while the second offers the best general compromise.]

Most first year nurses experience a bewildering diversity of opinions and attitudes on such matters as abortions, truthtelling, informed consent and death and dying. Because these diverse attitudes are often emotionally charged, and because our emotional responses are usually directed towards persons in such situations, it is easy to explain the great bulk of that diversity as due to individual personality differences. One is likely to hear psychological or sociological explanations for why someone behaves or believes in a certain way. "Dr. A once lost a patient through suicide when he told her she had breast cancer; that's why he doesn't tell his patients much." "Nurse B came from a large family that was very poor and she had an abusive mother; that's why she's so eager to assist in abortions." Or, one hears attitudes accounted for in terms of one's memberships in particular groups: "That social worker was raised a Catholic: that's why she works with retarded kids."

Now, these are perfectly ordinary and correct forms of explanation, of a very general casual sort. It is undeniable that a physician's early experiences with patients, especially if they are particularly satisfying or traumatic, can markedly influence later behavior. There's no question but that childhood experiences can predispose one towards a favorable or unfavorable stance for abortion on demand. There are certainly high

From *Kansas Nurse*, 55, October 1980, 4–5, 21–24. Reprinted with permission of the Kansas State Nurses' Association.

correlations between membership in certain religious groups and preference for careers of service to the handicapped. For their reasons for
these attitudes, beliefs and patterns of behavior, one is likely not to hear
the types of facts just cited. Rather, one is more likely to be given
explanations characterized by the presence of words like "best interests", "rights", "obligations." The physician in the earlier example is
likely to say, "It isn't in the best interests of most patients to be told
everything about their cases, because it is likely to unduly frighten
them." The nurse may say, "An unwanted child has a right not to be
born." The social worker might say, "We have a particular obligation to
provide loving care and opportunity for special children who are less
fortunate than ourselves." In other words, the types of explanations
which people give for their own attitudes, beliefs and behaviors frequently tend to be moral explanations, rather than psychological or
sociological ones. They seek to provide justification of attitudes, beliefs
and behaviors, and they then press others into agreement or into giving
defenses of contrary views.

The diversities which nurses encounter in patients and their families,
in physicians, in other nurses and other allied health personnel are
rooted in alternate views of humankind, not merely in individual person-
alities or group identities. We need an understanding of the philosophical and ethical presuppositions, not only of our own views but of those
with whom we disagree. This should enhance one's ability to deal effectively and productively with situations of ethical conflict to assist patients and their families in reaching and implementing ethically viable
decisions about their care, and to influence the policy-making processes
that go on in one's place of employment. Such understanding may also
be instrumental in helping to resolve in one's own mind the areas of
uncertainty and conflicting values that each of us occasionally confronts.

We shall briefly examine three images of humankind—views on both
the essence of what it is to be human and the associated principles of rights
and obligations. Next, we will connect each of these to one of the models
of the relationship between the patient and the physician that has been
developed in the literature on medical ethics in recent years. This will
permit us to examine those models for the best characterization of nurse/
physician and nurse/client interactions one would like to promote.

A.   THREE VIEWS OF HUMANITY AND ITS ETHIC

Three alternative approaches to the essence of being human seem to
be discernible in our culture.

The first image of humankind is the traditional, religious one; humans as creatures of God. In this view, the creator is thought of as the giver of moral law, intended to guide human conduct so as to conform with the divine will's purposes.

The value of each individual human being is measured in terms of the relation of creature to creator under the revealed purpose which the creator has intended for that creature. For humans this special relationship is sometimes captured under the rubric, "the sanctity of human life." This axiom, that each human life is sacred by virtue of being created by a supreme being, has a corollary. Each human life is equal in value to each other human life—that a person who has but a few moments to live is of no less value than one who has 70 years to live. A person who is handicapped and cannot service the needs of society is not less a human because of that. This is frequently the basic view behind individuals' opposition to abortion, whether of a normal fetus or one identified through amniocentesis as abnormal, and to mercy-killing or even to any instance of "benign neglect."

The second image of humanity is that of individualism. A human is viewed as essentially a creative being in a universe otherwise lacking value, purpose and meaning. Only individual human acts of valuing can generate value; there is no order of value which is either absolute or independent of individual human preferences. The enormous importance that this individualistic ethic places on the individual raises the autonomy of the individual to the highest point. What is in an individual's interest is a function of his or her set of preferences, goals and capacities. Thus the individual is in the best position to determine whether a proposed course of medical intervention is in his best interests. Since he is in the best position to know his own value preferences, capacity for pain and suffering, future business and social plans, and religious beliefs to evaluate the desirability of a particular treatment . . .(1)

With this view, and in contrast to the previous one, there is no basis for a waiver of informed consent, except when incapacity prevents one from exercising the power of choice autonomously. In the first view, there is an absolute and invariant standard of human conduct. In the second philosophical approach, there is no ethical standard, apart from my own values, against which to measure my behavior. My informed consent is thus essential to making an intervention right.

The third view of humanity is that the essence of being human lies within community. The value of the individual is expressed in his or her contribution to the whole. As in the second view, there is no divinely ordained moral order to which human behavior must conform. It is also the case that the moral order is not limited to, or even constituted by, the individual's self interest and acts of valuation.

Utilitarianism is the most common form of this ethic. The central point is that the individual's interests, to be legitimate, must accord with those of other individuals so as to maximize the general welfare. It is the general good that is to be served by individual choices and general policies. Where individual preferences do not conflict with the interests of others, individualistic and utilitarian ethics may not diverge. But where serving one individual's desires and wishes detracts from other's welfare, then, this ethic dictates the subordination of the individual's interests and desires.

B. THREE MODELS OF THE PATIENT-PHYSICIAN RELATIONSHIP

Three characterizations of the relationship between physician and patient have appeared in recent medical ethics literature. These are not the only ones. But they are useful to illustrate how medical ethics presupposes one or another view of the nature of humanity. The three models are the *Priestly, Contractual* and *Collegial* or *Team* model.

In the traditional religious view, human obligations in medical decision making are few and uncomplicated. This does not mean that they may be clearly and without difficulty applied to every case in a manner which yields a clear-cut decision. It does mean that the task of ethical assessment is simpler. There is little or no involvement of considerations about future consequences. There is a somewhat comforting aura of finitude that surrounds the decision-making process in medicine. There are limits to what is expected of us. Above given limits of wisdom and farsightedness we should not and need not aspire. One frequently encounters among those of this persuasion the admonition that one ought not to "play God", or try to relegislate morality in the light of increasing technical power.

Descriptions of the Priestly model vary according to the sympathies of the writer. One philosopher-physician, Howard Brody, writes, "In the 'Priestly Model' . . .the physician plays a role that is frankly paternalistic. The patient (who, we might say, has somehow 'sinned' by getting sick) comes for treatment, counsel, and comfort. The decisionmaking is placed in the physician's hands, and the patient who does not follow the doctor's orders is adding an even greater 'sin' on top of his illness . . . (A) chief sign of this model is the 'Speaking -as-a' syndrome: 'Speaking as your doctor, I feel that it is definitely time for you to undergo surgical sterilization.' The decision here is a moral, not a medical one; but the priest-doctor is presumed to have competence in both areas by virtue of his M.D. degree."(2) Clearly, this author doesn't have much patience with the priestly, paternalistic role into which doctors sometimes slip.

The physician may be relatively clear about the prescribed duties that are pertinent in a given case. The physician may have the clearest understanding of the empirical possibilities and contingencies. There may not be a conflict among the relevant moral rules that do apply. Here the physician is probably in the best position of those involved to make a valid judgement about the course of action that is required ethically. If there appear to be conflicting rules involved in a particular case, or if that case doesn't clearly fall under any moral prescription known to the physician, his or her limited expertise as a kind of amateur theological ethicist may be insufficient to provide clear guidance. In this situation, the physician, like the analog parish priest, would turn to the system of higher authorities which exist, in part, for the purpose of interpreting the moral law. But the search for higher authority is not likely to lead to the patient in this tradition.

There is another dimension to the patient-physician relationship which is illuminated under the Priestly model. It is not uncommon that a patient's diseases or disorders are partially due to behavior which is in the patient's control. Insofar as the religious ethic contains such admonitions as "The body is the temple of the soul" and thereby enjoins humans toward circumspection and moderation in consumption of food and drugs, in sexual activity, in rest and exercise, one whose disease stems directly or indirectly from a failure to behave in accordance with these injunctions may well be seen as having sinned. For a physician who has the point of view that so characterizes the patient's disease, the analogy between his role and that of the priest may recommend itself irresistibly. The patient, like the penitent sinner, suffers the pains of his wrongdoing and comes for a treatment which aims at rectifying his or her wrong as far as possible. The physician, like the priest, encounters the patient in a position of considerable potential to exert an influence that may alter the wrongdoer's ways. Even medical problems may traceable causally to the behavior of the patient are frequently viewed by patients as chastising visitations inflicted in retribution for wrongdoing. The analogy between physician and priest ultimately breaks down. But when viewed under the scope of traditional religious ethics, it illuminates why some feel most comfortable in the role of either patient or physician as characterized by the Priestly model.

The accompanying traditional view of the relationship of nurse to physician has been variously characterized as that of a handmaiden,(3) or a tool,(4) in the hands of the physician. The emphasis, or course, is on the nurse serving without questioning medical decisions. Various reminders of this subordinate status have existed in such practices as nurses rising when physicians (and even medical students) enter the room.(5) The common sociological explanation is that most nurses are female and most doctors are male. But this sociological fact receives additional explanation under the Priestly model. Being female, nurses are poor candidates for a paternalistic role in which religious authorities have been called "father" in recognition of their status as representatives of the divine masculine Personage. Finally, the meaning of the term "nurse" (one who nurtures, as a mother), characterizes the relationship between nurse and patient beyond that involved in the notion of physician's handmaiden or tool.

A second model of the patient/physician relation described in recent literature is the Contractual model.(6) This seeks to replace the paternalistic approach with recognition that inner-directed, highly independent individuals respond better to therapeutic regimens which they help to choose.(7) The "contract" is usually an implicit understanding between the patient and the physician concerning their mutual obligations and benefits which calls for a sharing of the decision making. Where there are significant, life-altering decisions to be made, the physician recognizes and respects the legitimacy of the patient's informed decision making in regards to value-laden matters. Once the general goals are agreed to, the patient accedes to the physician's superiority in making the technical decisions needed to implement them. Thus, the patient does not need to be kept informed on all the technical details, but expects to be consulted on decisions involving major courses of action, even when alternatives differ significantly on the probability of the desired outcome. For example, this view would recognize the legitimacy of a patient's preference for medical or radiation treatment over that of amputation, even when the latter had the greatest chance of saving life.

An important reservation that the physician makes on the Contractual model is the right not to enter into the contract if the patient's wishes would, if implemented by the physician, force the latter to violate his or her own moral values. Thus, a physician would not be obligated to respond positively to a patient's request for an abortion if that ran counter to her/his deeply held convictions. A physician would be obligated to bow to a patient's wishes to increase the dosage of morphine for otherwise intractable pain, even if doing so increased the risk of a somewhat shortened life span. (There is some dispute among proponents of the Contractual view on whether a physician retains the right to withhold a standard medical service, such as abortion, on personal moral grounds if he or she represents the patient's only realistic alternative.)

The Contractual model appears to hold considerable attraction for nursing and its aspirations. First, it provides a recognition, in the principles of individualism, of the importance of providing nurses the same rights and respect captured for patients and physicians in the model. Extrapolating the model to nursing, we see that the nurse enters into a tacit agreement with both physician and patients (or clients) in which the rights and obligations of each party are recognized and respected by the others. Nurses and physicians accept that patients have the right to determine the major objectives of medical intervention aiming at the general ends of the patient. Physicians and patients will accord to nurses primary authority in determining the details of nursing care. Second, just as physicians reserve the right not to provide even standard medical treatments to patients where providing those treatments would be morally repugnant, so the nurse would seem, on the Contractual model, to reserve the right to refuse to participate in actions that would violate strongly held personal values. Finally, insofar as the mutual agreement between all parties is to cover benefits as well as rights, nursing finds in the Contractual model and individualistic ethics a basis for negotiating improvements in compensation, working conditions and other areas of needed reform.

The final model considered here is more closely coordinated with the image of humans as essentially social beings. Specific obligations of a moral character arise out of a general duty to seek to maximize the welfare and happiness of the greatest number of individuals possible. As indicated earlier, the status of individual interests and desires is one of conditional legitimacy—the condition being that they not be pursued to the detriment of others. The Team model (which has been called the Collegial model by others(8)) suggests that the physician and patient, rather than seeing themselves in a relationship suggestive of bargaining and legalism, see themselves as colleagues. They are coinvestigators pursuing the common goal of identifying and eliminating the illness and restoring the health of the patient. This is a relationship characterized by mutual trust and harmony, with an equality, if not coincidence, of value considerations. It aims at the utilitarian's maximization of welfare. Individuals are better off in active, participating roles even as patients than when forced to suffer either the passivity of the Priestly model or the rather limited decision-making functions of the Contractual model. The possibilities of involving the patient as a colleague have recently been eloquently explored by Norman Cousins.(9) John Gunther(10) has also provided a moving account of how, in the special situation of parental colleagueship, the parents of a young cancer patient participated actively and constructively in the planning of his treatment. And Renee Fox(11) has recounted the active participation and contribution of patients in kidney research programs.

The potential of the Team model to transform nurse/physician relations has not received the kind of attention in the public press as has its power for the physician/patient relationship. But it is evident that, among colleagues who accord to one another an equality of dignity and respect and who acknowledge shared responsibility and accountability for their actions, there is a greater likelihood of consensus as to mutual ends and means. This does not appeal necessarily to a consensus model of diagnostic or therapeutic decision making. Each involved party can be accorded the right and responsibility to have primary input and final say over that portion of the case where his or her expertise is most relevant. At the same time, the mutuality of respect and the sense of common purpose which members of the team accord to one another creates an atmosphere in which the checks and balances of constructive criticism and review can operate in a wholesome and non-threatening way.

It may be that the circumstances and stage of the case will dictate that some one member of the team fulfill the role of captain, the one charged with generating the major decisions for that stage of the case. That captaincy, however, is not automatically determined by rank or title or degree, but rather by the character and stage of the case. The physician is only one member of the team, whose ascendency comes at the points of diagnosis and interpretation, perhaps again at the point of treatment implementation. One of the chief functions of the physician, however, is to issue an accurate set of conditionals: "If you want to maximize your chances of surviving this throat cancer, then present statistics indicate you will do so only by a combination of surgery and radiation therapy; if it is more important to you to lead a relatively normal next few months than to maximize your chances of surviving five years, then radiation therapy alone is indicated," and so on. But the physician who diagnoses may be neither the one who operates nor the one who delivers radiation therapy. And in terms of planning daily postoperative care, the importance of any physician may be vanishingly small in contract to that of the nurse, the physical therapist and the dietician. And the ultimate decision as between the conditionals offered by the physician may be made by the patient or by the patient's proxy, who thereby determines the points and times of the ascendancy of other members of the team to its captaincy. Rather than representing each of these individuals as entering into a contractual relationship that is characterized by potentially competing self-interests (as in the Contractual model), and rather than automatically deferring to the physician's authority, the Team model characterizes the mutual relationship as centering around a set of common values and goals adopted by the members of the team in consenting to participate in the joint venture.

C. LIMITATIONS AND RELATIVE MERITS OF THE THREE MODELS

There are several reasons why the Priestly model is the least satisfactory of the three. First, it presupposes a religious orientation that is not universal, even among believers. The system of specially appointed protectors of morality is not common to a sufficient portion of religions and religious sects to make that mode of behavior on the part of the physician comfortable for most patients. This is especially true when one is increasingly unlikely to have the same physician throughout one's life and thus unlikely to develop a sense of that individual being thoroughly knowledgeable and wise about one's needs and individual quirks. Second, the model runs counter to so many other movements and trends (e.g., the patients' rights movement) as to be something of an anachronism. Third, it is widely and increasingly perceived as derogatory and demeaning of the nurse, and even as promoting an unhealthy image of the doctor whose "status is a function of the vacuum created by the nurse's low self-esteem".(12) Certainly it is less than ideal as a model to be emulated by a profession working to improve its own image. Its major merit is to serve as a reminder that there are patients who need a paternalistic approach, even to the point of believing that the physician is in total and complete charge.

The Contractual model, of course, will not work as well with that type of patient if he or she is forced into the position of actively processing information and deciding between alternative courses of therapy. However, it is possible to avoid this consequence by noting that it is certainly legitimate in the individualistic approach (although not very laudatory) for one to assign to a proxy (family member, friend, physician, nurse or whoever is willing to take it) the decision making function. This is probably what goes on when a patient, confronted by a doctor who is carefully explaining the options, comes up with, "whatever you say, Doctor." That is a patient who is attempting to contract with the physician to play according to the Priestly model's rules.

A deeper flaw of the Contractual model stemming from its roots in individualism is that it virtually capitulates to a kind of relativism of morals, in which each individual is his own source of morality and any one individual's ethic is as good as any other. The Contractual model does not impose any general goals for the negotiating parties. Each is free to lay down his or her limits as to what services to offer or withhold on moral grounds and the patient is free to elect the least promising alternative on the basis of whim or even of a desire to end life. This model provides no incentive or even justification for the kind of counseling that can bolster a flagging spirit and transmit the resolve to seek the longer, more painful therapy which has the better chance of success. In short, the Contractual model is essentially amoral and can work well, but to the detriment of the patient. Nor is the health care professional immune to this sort of effect. Provided that what the patient elects is not inherently offensive to the moral sensitivities of the physician or nurse, the latter have no basis in the model for refusing to cooperate or even for advising the patient that they believe his choice to be ill-advised. To object would presuppose some standard of value external to the patient's own choice-making and individualism denies that possibility.

While the Team model with the presupposition of a utilitarian ethic seems to have a remedy for many of these foregoing defects, it too is not without its problems. First and perhaps foremost, there are extraordinary interpersonal problems that can arise in seeking to implement the Team model among professionals who have been used to other approaches. Physicians seem notoriously inclined to regard the increased participation of the nurse as an usurpation of their responsibility and authority and the transfer of comprehensive functions as not a delegation but a surrender of them.(13) This potential for a sense of professional encroachment is increasingly familiar to nurses as they view the development and spread of Physician's Assistant programs. It would seem that a precondition for the successful application of the Team model would be the successful negotiation of the division of labors and responsibilities by the prospective members of each team.(14) A second source of resistance to the team approach can be the individual nurse who may be unprepared for the increased leadership, responsibility and participation in decision-making functions. A third source of conflict in implementing the Team model is the fact that economic differences among team members may be greater than seem justified to individuals who have come to regard one another as colleagues and as increasingly equal in interprofessional status.(15) Finally, a major source of resistance may be encountered in the patient who is accustomed to conducting all negotiations through the physician. It is clear that the education and realignment of all members of the team will be a major task. Insofar as present structuring of medicine and health care delivery does not make for constancy of association among relatively small groups, that education and retraining may well be ongoing.

The possibilities of opting effectively for the Team model seem at present rather limited, restricted to relatively small groups that are thrown into close and continual professional proximity. Where those conditions can be met, and there is successful negotiation of the many issues involving shared responsibility and accountability, it can be an enormously pleasant and rewarding form of professional interaction. The Contractual model perhaps offers the best general compromise. It provides for the Priestly model, where tradition and personality type make that the most effective mode, without endorsing the general applicability of that kind of physician-centered structure. The Priestly model will continue (although perhaps with decreasing frequency) to be encountered by the nurse. The tensions between the three models are lived out by all nurses. It is hoped that this discussion will enable the nurse to recognize her situation(s) and better change them for her patient's and her own well-being.

ENDNOTES

1. Charles Montagne, "Informed Consent and the Dying Patient," Yale Law Review 83 (July 74), 1646.

2. Howard Brody, Ethical Decisions in Medicine; Boston: Little, Brown, 1976, p. 31.

3. Cf. Larry Churchill, "Ethical Issues of a Profession in Transition," AJN 77 (May 77), 873.

4. James Gustafson, "Mongolism, Parental Desires and the Right to Life," Perspectives in Biology and Medicine 16 (Sum 73), 548.

5. Churchill, op. cit.

6. Robert Veach, "Models for Ethical Medicine in a Revolutionary Age," HCR 2, No. 3 (June 72), 5–7.

7. Rue L. Cromwell, Earl C. Butterheid, Frances M. Brayheld & John J. Curry, Acute Myocardial Infarction: Reaction and Recovery; St. Louis: Mosby, 1977.

8. Veatch, op cit. Brody, op cit.

9. Norman Cousins, "Anatomy of an Illness," NEJM (23 Dec 76), 1458–1463. Id., Anatomy of an Illness as Perceived by the Patient; NY: Norton, 1979. Id., The Healing Heart: Antidote to Pain and Helplessness; NY: Norton, 1983.]

10. John Gunther, Death Be Not Proud; NY: Harper & Brothers, 1949.

11. Renee C. Fox, Experiment Perilous; Glencoe: Free Press, 1959.

12. Churchill, op cit.

13. Barbara Bates, "Doctor and Nurse: Changing Roles and Relations," NEJM 283, No. 3 (16 July 70), 129.

14. Shirley Smoyak. "Problems in Interprofessional Relations," Bulletin of the New York Academy of Medicine, 53 (1977), 51–9.

15. Veatch, op. cit.

CHAPTER 15

WHOSE AUTONOMY IS AT STAKE?

Nora K. Bell

[An analysis of the Tuma case shows the physician acted unethically and illegally. This was not faced by the courts which sidestepped the issue of informed consent. The court protected the physician privilege and ignored patient autonomy.]

Jolene Tuma, R.N., a nursing instructor, was caring for a leukemia patient who was scheduled for chemotherapy which the patient's physician had told her was her only hope for survival. The patient had fought her leukemia for 12 years with faith in God. Tuma discussed with the patient the latter's condition and background. They discussed alternative treatments such as chaparral and laetrile. The patient asked Tuma to return in the evening and discuss these things with the family. Tuma started the chemotherapy. The patient called her family and asked them not to tell the physician for it could cause Tuma trouble. The daughter-in-law called the physician anyway who thus knew about the meeting but did nothing to stop it nor did he talk further with the patient nor with Tuma. After discussion with the family, the parties decided to continue the chemotherapy. Later that month, hospital personnel called the Board of Nursing of the State of Idaho complaining that Tuma had interfered with the physician-patient relationship. Tuma had her license expended for six months for interfering in a physician-patient relationship.

In my view, that decision, later reversed by the Supreme Court of Idaho, was both morally and pragmatically unacceptable.

The Idaho Supreme Court said that Ms. Tuma's license could not be suspended because the Board of Nursing's rules and regulations did not adequately warn that interfering with a physician-patient relationship was unprofessional conduct. This ruling sidesteps, however understandably, what I take to be the larger moral issues in question.

Several ethical issues in health care delivery run together in this case.

As I see it, these include the patient's rights, especially those deriving from the requirements of informed consent; the appropriateness of the physician's actions; the appropriateness of the nurse's actions; and the limits of professionals' "rights" to access to and treatment of their patients.

Given this range of issues, and given that an obligation to one's patient is central to the ethics of all health professions, I believe that the charge against the nurse was both misleading and incongruous. It was misleading because it did not address the wrong done to the patient. If anything, it suggested that a wrong was done to the physician.

What should have been at issue here were the patient's rights, not an infringement of the physician's "right" to his patient. It was also misleading in that it served as a smokescreen for the physician's apparent failure to meet the consent requirements.

The charge is incongruous because implicit in the charge is the notion that the doctor-patient relationship is primary. In most states, laws or conventions regarding physician privilege tend to support this notion. However, if, in fact, the doctor-patient relationship is primary, it was the doctor's duty to inform and advise his patient concerning alternative therapies. Yet, he apparently didn't.

If the charge was intended to establish that the nurse infringed on the "right" of the physician to his patient, it was misstated. The charge should have been that the nurse exceeded the scope of her authority. But if the intent of the charge was to focus on the nature of the doctor-patient relationship and to suggest that the quality of it was impaired by Ms. Tuma's actions, then it requires closer scrutiny.

To couch the charge in such terms as the nurse "disrupted," "impaired," or "interfered with" the doctor-patient relationship is to suggest that the relationship was previously a good or proper one. Certainly, one must ask, Was the nurse's action wrong? But another question in this case is, Was this a good doctor-patient relationship, one that the nurse could "impair"?

Answers to these questions and the explanation of my objections to the original decision require a partial analysis of the ethics of consent and the implications of consent requirements for the nature of the doctor-patient relationship.

A. INFORMED CONSENT

The notion of informed consent is neither new nor novel. The principle underlying the giving of free and adequately informed consent was announced as early as 1914, when it was ruled that "every human being of adult years and sound mind has a right to determine what shall be done with his own body."(1)

As a philosopher, I argue that the principle of informed consent affirms individual autonomy, the patient's rights to be master of his own fate—in sum, it's an affirmation of respect for persons. The principle of informed consent must be understood as asserting that the person is not merely a passive subject, a thing to be acted on at the physician's discretion.(2)

There is philosophical precedent for holding such a principle. Put in the Kantian idiom, the requirement of informed consent affirms that persons are ends in themselves. For Kant, to respect persons means to acknowledge that there is a difference between things, which have only conditional worth or worth for us as a means to some end, and persons, whose existence in itself has some absolute worth.(3)

To insist upon a respect for persons means to acknowledge oneself and others as capable of self-determination rather than as determined by others. It is to insist that in matters involving a person's bodily or personal integrity, the requirements of informed consent are always to be regarded as relevant and binding. Informed consent is essential precisely because one's worth as a human overrides anything that would allow one to be treated as a thing in order to gain some perceived "good" as a consequence.

When health care providers affirm the moral legitimacy of a principle that champions individual autonomy—even if they are only succumbing to convention by engaging in such a practice; they acknowledge that the provider-patient relationship is essentially consensual. Conceived of in this way, consent requirements mimic contract requirements between two individuals—in this case, between patient and physician.

While some prefer to speak of the proper model for doctor-patient relationships as contractual, the term seems far too legalistic.(4,5)

Though the requirements of informed consent have been legalized to some extent, "consensual" seems to better capture the intended moral nature of the relationship. In either case, however, failure to meet the conditions grounding the relationship voids that relationship.

Because seeking another's consent carries the notion of truth-telling, hence trust, and because it underscores respect for one's right to be self-determined, the notion of informed consent seems to generate a duty on the part of the physician to apprise his patient of all data relevant to making a decision on the proposed treatment. In Canterbury v. Spence, the court stated, "True consent to what happens to oneself is the informed exercise of a choice, and that entails an opportunity to evaluate knowledgeably the options available. . . . From these almost axiomatic considerations springs . . . a duty to impart information which the patient has every right to expect."(6)

In order for one to exercise his right to be master of his own fate and to feel that he has made an intelligent decision regarding a proposed treatment, a patient must be able to trust that some minimum obligation accrues to the physician to convey adequate information and that the physician will fulfill this obligation. Such trust "grounds" the consent requirement.

Certainly, it is very difficult in some cases to determine whether one is bound by the moral rule governing informed consent. What constitutes being of "sound mind"? What counts as "adequate" information? What is the extent of "information significant enough for a reasonable man" to refuse treatment? All are vague and debatable criteria. Despite this, if we are to hold to the principles underlying the notion of informed consent, the presumption must be in favor of the patient and against exceptions to the requirements of informed consent.

This all suggests a radical departure from the traditional, paternalistic model of physician-patient relationships.

Paternalism is both logically and morally incompatible with the rule of informed consent. The only cases where paternalism could be justified and where securing consent is morally and legally unnecessary are emergency situations and situations in which the patient has specifically relinquished the right to informed consent by asking not to be told certain things. The duty in all other cases is to seek both full disclosure and the patient's understanding of the proposed treatment.

From the ethnicist's point of view, the physician who chooses the paternalistic model is acting on the belief that his or her judgments and interest are of greater worth than those of the patient. The very possibility that the physician's judgement may be impaired by a strong desire for a certain outcome ought to strengthen the resolve to adhere to the principles of informed consent. To do otherwise is to disavow, at least implicitly, the right of persons (including the physician) to be self-determined.

B.   IMPLICATIONS OF TUMA

The case of nursing instructor Tuma makes a mockery of informed consent for several reasons.

As I noted earlier, determining when a physician has provided his patient with "information adequate for an intelligent decision" is fraught with difficulties. In the Tuma case, it could be argued that the physician really had no more obligation to tell his patient about Laetrile and herbal cures than he did to tell her about voodoo or the belief that eating blueberries cures cancer. After all, if other possible "cures" are not considered by the physician to be legitimate therapy options, could one expect a physician to describe them or to believe that knowledge of them is necessary for making an informed decision about the proposed treatment?

But the fact that this patient asked about alternative therapies and was uncertain about the prescribed treatment, a treatment decided on by her son and the physician, suggests that she really had not had a chance to discuss her beliefs and her anxieties with her physician. The doctor-patient relationship, in this case, appears to have been inadequate at least insofar as the patient was unable to discuss with her physician, in a way that she could understand, the effectiveness or ineffectiveness of therapies she thought to be viable options.

Whether the physician's judgment as to the value of certain of these alternative therapies was justified or not, certainly the moral force of the rule of informed consent required that he seek to uncover and quiet her fears about chemotherapy as well as to acknowledge that the decision lay ultimately in the hands of the patient.

Finally, informed consent cannot be construed as growing out of an agreement between a physician and the son of a mentally competent adult patient. One cannot consent for another who is capable of giving her own consent any more than one can unilaterally give away the rights of another. Rather than obtaining consent from an informed patient, it seems that this physician relied on an informed, or acquiescent, son to pressure the patient.

Given such circumstances, I maintain that the doctor/patient relationship was impaired in the first instance, not by the nurse, but by the doctor himself. Whatever relationship did exist between this patient and her physician was founded in distrust. For the physician and the patient's son, it was a distrust that she could be relied upon, given the full information, to make a sound judgment in her own best interest. Surely this cannot be the ground of a good relationship—one that someone else could "impair."

The bilateral trust that must underlie the relationship demanded by the principles of informed consent was broken when the doctor failed to ensure that his patient understood and was informed about the proposed therapy—when he failed to affirm her right to be self-determined.

Having lamented the lack of informed consent and the absence of a good physician-patient relationship, one must still ask whether what the nursing instructor did in this case was right.

Clearly, the moral principles underlying the rule of informed consent weighs as heavily on the nurse as they do on the physician. Surely a commitment to patient autonomy entails a responsibility to ensure the patient's comprehension of a proposed therapy. One's inclination might be to insist that the nurse's moral duty to her patient overrides prudential considerations. It is easy to say, given this duty, that the nursing instructor did the right thing.

However, affirming patient autonomy can be achieved in a number of ways. The admonition to physicians against allowing individual interests to impede judgments applies not to physicians alone. Patient advocacy does not require that members of various health professions establish their own autonomy.

If a nurse feels that a patient lacks adequate information for understanding his or her therapy, patient advocacy requires no more than going to the physician with the request that more detailed information be given to the patient or letting the physician know that the patient seeks advice on alternative forms of therapy.

The nurse can express her own autonomy by refusing to administer treatment until the patient's requests have been met.

In the event that a physician refused to acknowledge either the patient's or the nurse's request, then surely patient advocacy would require that the nurse seek to provide the patient with the information required by the rule of informed consent. This would not be exceeding the limits of her authority—it would be her duty as required by the principles implicit in informed consent.

Establishing the limits of the autonomy of the different health professions is quite a different matter, one not appropriately discussed here. With respect to the case in question, two points seem in order. First, patients' rights should not fall before disputes over professional boundaries. And second, inasmuch as the nursing instructor was not charged with exceeding the limits of her authority, but with disturbing what seems to have been an inadequate relationship, the charge was untenable.

ENDNOTES

1. Scholendorff vs. Society of N.Y. Hospital, 211 NY 125, 129, 105 NE 92, 92, 1914.

2. Paul Ramsey, The Patient as Person; New Haven, CT: Yale, 1970, pp. 2–11.

3. Immanuel Kant, Foundations of the Metaphysics of Morals; Indianapolis, IN: Liberal Arts Press, 1959, p. 428.

4. Howard Brody, Ethical Decisions in Medicine; Boston: Little, Brown, 1976, pp. 31–46.

5. Thomas S. Szasz and Marc H. Hollender, "A Contribution to the Philosophy of Medicine—The Basic Models of the Doctor/Patient Relationship," Archives of Internal Medicine 97, No. 5 (May 56), 585–592.

6. Canterbury vs. Spence, 464 F 2d 772 (D.C. Cir. 1972).

FOR FURTHER READING

Elsie L. Bandman, "How Much Dare You Tell Your Patient?," RN 41, No. 8 (Aug 78), 39–41.

Joseph L. Bejsovec, et al., "More on the Tuma Case," NO 26, No. 1 (Jan 78), 8–9.

Vernice Ferguson, "Informed Consent: Given the Facts," Nursing Mirror 153, No. 1 (1 July 81), 35–36.

———, "The Tuma Case: Other Options," NO 26, No. 3 (Mar 78), 142–143.

William J. Gargaro, "Informed Consent," Cancer Nursing 1, No. 6 (Dec 78), 467–468.

———, "Informed Consent: A Specific Case," Cancer Nursing 1, No. 4 (Aug 78), 329–330.

Joanne Comi McCloskey, et al., "Ethics: Overview, Debate, Viewpoints," pp. 705–764 in Current Issues in Nursing ed McCloskey and Helen K. Grace; Boston: Blackwell Scientific Publications, 1981.

Hildegard E. Peplau, et al., "Feedback on 'The Right to Inform'," NO 25, No. 12 (Dec 77), 738–740.

Teresa Stanley, "Ethical Reflections on the Tuma Case: Is it Part of the Nurse's Role to Advise on Alternate Forms of Therapy or Treatment?," pp. 717–726 in Current Issues in Nursing ed Joanne Comi McCloskey and Helen K. Grace; Boston: Blackwell, 1982.

———, "Is it Ethical to give hope to a dying person?," Nursing Clinics of North America 14, No. 1 (Mar 79), 69–80.

Jolene L. Tuma, "Professional Misconduct?," NO 25, No. 9 (Sep 77), 546.

Gerald R. Winslow, "From Loyalty to Advocacy: A New Metaphor for Nursing," HCR 14, No. 3 (June 84), 32–40.

Jo Ann T. Vahey, "Implications of the Tuma Decision," NO 27, No. 7 (July 79), 438–439.

SECTION VI
RESEARCH

CHAPTER 16

ETHICS AND NURSING RESEARCH

Sara T. Fry

[Fry considers ethical principles and issues in research. The first includes respect for persons, beneficence, and justice. The second includes moral justification for research, informed consent, selection of subjects, and risk/benefits. When nursing research meets these standards, nursing is improved through research.]

Experimentation involving human subjects is as old as that of nursing care itself. Throughout history, every society has had health workers who, by one means or another, have attempted to devise better ways to prevent illness, restore the sick to health or rehabilitate those suffering from chronic disease. Over the years, certain rules of conduct have emerged from these various attempts to improve the health of one's fellow citizens.

Some of these rules have been incorporated into codes of research ethics with particular focus on the use of human subjects in research. Beginning with the Nuremberg Code of 1947, to the Declaration of Helsinki adopted by the World Medical Association in 1964, and even the 1975 American Nurses' Association "Human Rights Guidelines for Nurses in Clinical and Other Research," codes have consisted of rules that guide investigators in their work.

In recent times, however, it has been recognized that rules of conduct often conflict with one another and sometimes prove difficult to apply to specific situations. Addressing this problem, the National Commission for the Protection of Human Subjects of Biomedical and Behavioral Research issued a statement of broad principles as a basis for the formulation and interpretation of specific rules in the conduct of research involving human subjects. This statement, "The Belmont Report," presents three general ethical principles to "assist scientists, subjects, review-

---

From *Virginia Nurse,* Summer 1982. Reprinted with permission of the Virginia Nurses' Association.

ers, and interested citizens to understand the ethical issues inherent in research involving human subjects."(1)

The purpose of this presentation is to analyze these ethical principles and demonstrate how they influence our deliberation of ethical problems or issues which arise in research involving human subjects. Starting with a discussion of ethical principles in research, I will then analyze specific issues in research focusing on how principles of ethics influence these issues in nursing research or research designed to improve the practice of nursing.

A. ETHICAL PRINCIPLES RELEVANT TO RESEARCH

"The Belmont Report" states, "basic ethical principles refer to those general judgments that serve as a basic justification for the many particular ethical prescriptions and evaluations of human actions."(2) This statement means that basic ethical principles provide a foundation for second-order principles and rules. These principles may also serve, along with rules, as action guides to concrete situations.(3) Although "The Belmont Report" notes that there may be many ethical principles, it identifies three basic, comprehensive principles relevant to research involving human subjects: the principles of respect for persons, beneficence, and justice.

Respect for Persons

Respect for persons contains at least two basic convictions: first, that individuals should be treated as autonomous agents; and second, that persons with diminished autonomy are entitled to protection.(4) We think of an autonomous person as one who is capable of deliberating about personal goals and of acting under the direction of this deliberation.(5) As nurse researchers, we respect autonomy by seriously considering the opinions and choices of autonomous persons while not, at the same time, obstructing their actions unless they are harmful to others. If we deny a person the freedom to act on his judgments or withhold information necessary to make judgments, we show a lack of respect for autonomous agents.

However the nurse must recognize when human subjects are not capable of self-determination. The capacity for self-determination is relative to maturity, chronological age, the presence or absence of illness, mental disability or other social situations that restrict a person's liberty to be self-determining. Respect for persons requires that researchers recognize when persons lack the capacity to act autonomously and therefore are entitled to protection.

Respect for persons also requires that the subjects of research be voluntary participants. They should have necessary information concerning the risks and benefits of the research, and in certain social situations, receive added consideration as to their social capacity to make an adequate, informed consent to participate in the research study.

Beneficence

The second ethical principle important to research is that of beneficence. "The Belmont Report" points out that beneficence is understood as a principle of obligation or duty to (1) not harm others and (2) maximize possible benefits and minimize possible harms that might occur in research.(6) Meeting both of these obligations always poses certain challenges for the researcher. Sometimes it is justifiable to seek certain benefits even though certain risks are involved or to decide when benefits should be foregone because of the risks involved in the research.(7)

Research that poses minimal or more than minimal risk to the research subject presents a difficult ethical problem when it is performed for the benefit of others. In other words, where does one set the ceiling on the amount of risk we allow research subjects to be exposed to for the greater good of society's health or the health benefit to a particular population? Although the principle of beneficence covers several different aspects of research—direct benefit to a particular research subject, indirect benefit to others outside the research protocol, and benefit to society's health in general—it is always difficult to determine which benefit carries the most weight in research decisions.

Justice

The third principle is that of justice. We understand this principle to mean that equals should be treated equally, or that there is a fair manner in which social burdens and benefits ought to be allocated.(8) In research settings, the principle of justice dictates how the selection of research subjects is made; that is, are some classes of persons being selected for the research study because of their easy availability, because they are a captive audience, so to speak, or is their selection truly related to the problem under consideration in the research study? The question of justice also surfaces in the use of persons in research when it is unlikely that they will ever be beneficiaries of the research results.

B.   ETHICAL ISSUES IN RESEARCH

All three of the ethical principles: respect for persons, beneficence, and justice—gain significance in the consideration of specific issues that frequently arise in research involving human subjects.(9) Some of these issues are (1) the justification for research, (2) informed consent, (3) the selection of subjects of research and (4) the risk/benefit assessment of research.

Moral Justification for Research

Prior to the 1970's, very little attention was devoted to the moral justification of research involving human subjects. Most of the codes of research ethics simply assumed that research would be performed in part "for the sake of the knowledge to be gained" or "for the good of society."(10) Since the traditional ethic of health care has been that of a patient benefit ethic—from Hippocrates to modern times—this emphasis on knowledge for the good of society has been questioned. A major result has been the development of federal regulations for the conduct of research involving human subjects including guidelines to meet ethical requirements for research.

Professional groups, such as the American Nurses' Association, have also developed codes of ethics to help guide members who engage in research. In 1975, the ANA affirmed the profession's obligation to support the advancement of scientific knowledge toward the achievement of improved and nursing practice and better patient care in the "Human Rights Guidelines for Nurses in Clinical and other Research." By establishing these guidelines, the ANA accepted a commitment to support two sets of human rights. One set is concerned with the rights of qualified nurses (those with research preparation) to engage in research and to have access to resources necessary for implementing scientific investigations. The other set is concerned with the human rights of all persons who are recipients of health care services or are participants in research performed by investigators whose studies impinge on the patient care provided by nurses.(11)

In establishing the "Human Rights Guidelines," the nursing profession acknowledged the social and technological changes that have altered nursing and nursing practice in the last decade and the ethical problems that have accompanied these changes. This important professional document also recognizes that the relationship of trust between patient and nurse is an important value which influences the practice of nursing. In research contexts, the trust relationship between subject and investigator may even require the investigator to assume special obligations to safeguard the subject. Thus, it appears that the nursing profession considers the protection of human rights—especially the right to self-determination—to be an important factor in the justification of research.

Interestingly enough, the ANA "Human Rights Guidelines" acknowledge that the rights of individuals "are of necessity counterbalanced by actions and activities designed for the common good of collective man."(12) Many public health measures practiced today are a result of research seeking ways to treat and control disease for the common good. Accordingly, the "Humans Rights Guidelines" note that "personal rights may give way to collective rights for the benefit of society as a whole."(13) Although the nurse's primary responsibility is always to client care and safety—in other words, a protect-the-patient-from-harm ethic—it is conceivable that the balancing of moral responsibilities may create conflict for the nurse researcher. The nurse is obligated to protect the human rights of patients in research endeavors, yet the "Human Rights Guidelines" state clearly that the nurse has the additional obligation to "support the accrual of knowledge that broadens the scientific underpinnings of nursing practice and the delivery of nursing services."(14)

It seems that there is a decided consequentalistic twist to the moral justification of scientific research conducted by the nurse. Emphasis on the common good of collective man suggests that nursing can preempt the needs of individuals for the needs of larger populations once the nurse determines that the benefit to larger populations carries greater weight than the benefit to the individual research subject. Balancing both of these obligations—respect for basic human rights and benefit in the form of improved nursing services—may thus prove difficult in the quest for nursing knowledge. This is a problem that inevitably tests the moral justification of research studies to improve the practice of nursing.

Informed Consent

The principle of respect for persons requires that research subjects be given "The opportunity to choose what shall or shall not happen to them."(15) Research subjects are provided this opportunity when adequate disclosure standards for informed consent are included in the research protocol. In "The Belmont Report," three elements essential to adequate informed consent are noted: information, comprehension, and voluntariness.

Information: In order for the research subject to have adequate information, the researcher must disclose information pertaining to the research procedure, its purposes, any risks and anticipated benefits, alternative procedures for therapy, and a statement offering the subject the opportunity to ask questions or to withdraw at any time from the research.(16) The "Final Regulations Amending Basic DHHS Policy for the Protection of Human Research Subjects," dated January 26, 1981, also note that adequate informed consent should include a statement describing the extent, if any, to which confidentiality of records identifying the subject will be maintained; also, whom to contact pertaining to research subject questions or research related injury.(17) In research involving minimal risk, there must also be explanation as to whether any compensation or any medical treatments are available if injury occurs and what they consist of.

In the "Human Rights Guidelines," the element of information is included within provisions for adequate disclosure. They state, "the person's consent must be . . . without deception being practiced upon the subject. Should the research design require some degree of concealment of the true purpose or methodology of the study, the design must also provide for subsequent disclosure of the nature of the concealment and the rationale for incorporating secrecy as part of the procedure."(18) But the interesting question to ask concerning information supplied to research participants is how much information is enough? One of the standards frequently resorted to, especially in malpractice law, is the standard of reasonable person. In other words, the researcher is required to "reveal the information that reasonable persons would wish to know in order to make a decision regarding their care."(19) Thus, the strongest ethical principle operating in informed consent, particularly where information is concerned, is that of autonomy. Because human subjects are autonomous persons with all the entitlements that autonomous persons possess, researchers have a moral duty to disclose information relative to the research subjects' needs.(20)

Comprehension: However, information is not the only element in informed consent. The manner and context in which information is conveyed is equally important in order for comprehension to take place. Research subjects must be allowed the time for consideration of information and the time to ask questions. I must point out, however, that a subject's ability to understand or comprehend is a function of one's competence to understand; also, "a person is competent if and only if that person can make decisions based on rational reasons."(21) This definition of competency "entails that a person must be able to understand a therapy or research procedure, must be able to weigh its risk and benefits, and must be able to make a decision in the light of such knowledge and through such abilities, even if the person chooses not to utilize the information."(22)

When competence severely limits one's comprehension of information provided by the researcher, the principle of respect for persons requires the giving of additional opportunities to choose to the extent they are able, whether or not they want to participate in research.(23) Heeding the principle of respect for persons may even mean that permission of others authorized to act in a person's best interests is necessary in order to protect the subject from harm. An example would be the permission of parents in research using children. Other classes of subjects falling into this group include mentally disabled patients, the terminally ill or comatose patients.

In the ANA "Human Rights Guidelines" the principle of respect for persons is acknowledged where "the informed consent of parents and legal guardians must be obtained for investigations that involve minors or individuals judged to be legally incompetent to handle their own affairs."(24) The principle is further upheld by the provision, "In instances in which these subjects have the capacity to comprehend the implication of the proposed activity they should also be asked to give their consent. In this case consent supplements rather than supplants that of the parent or other legal agent."(25)

Voluntariness: The element of voluntariness is also essential to informed consent. This element is so important that an agreement to participate in research constitutes a valid consent only if voluntarily given, free of coercion and undue influence by other persons or institutions. Again, the principle of respect for persons is the main ethical principle guiding this provision. The very notion of voluntariness connotes the ability to choose one's own goals and to be able to choose among several goals when offered a choice of options.(26) As the Human Rights Guidelines point out, "the person's consent must be voluntarily given without overt or covert coercion being used and without deception being practiced upon the subject."(27)

These three elements—information, comprehension, and voluntariness—comprise informed consent in nursing as well as all research involving human subjects. No informed consent is valid without all elements; and no research involving human subjects is ethically acceptable without valid, informed consent.

Selection of Research Subjects

A third ethical issue in research revolves around the selection of research subjects. Unfortunately, codes of research ethics have had precious little to say concerning this topic. It is, however, an important issue in experimentation when we consider two major studies conducted during this century.

The first is the study of mentally retarded children at Willowbrook State Hospital, Staten Island, New York and their susceptibility to infectious hepatitis.(28) In 1956, physicians at Willowbrook began studies on infectious hepatitis, a disease that was very prevalent at the institution. Children admitted into a special research unit were injected with infected serum to produce hepatitis "to gain a better understanding of the disease and if possible, to develop methods of immunizing against hepatitis."(29)

The second research study prompting ethical debate is the Tuskegee Syphilis Study. This study was begun in 1932 in Macon County, Alabama by the U.S. Public Health service. Its purpose was "to determine the natural course of untreated, latent syphilis in black males."(30) Four hundred syphilitic men were studied and 200 uninfected men served as study controls. Even after penicillin was widely available as the preferred treatment for syphilis, however, study participants did not receive therapy. In fact, the study was not halted until 1972 and then only after reports of the study appeared in the national press. By that time, "seventy-four of the test subjects were still alive; at least twenty-eight, but perhaps more than 100 had died directly from advanced syphilitic lesions."(31)

Many questions have been raised about these two research studies: questions about the protection of incompetent persons (the mentally retarded, children, and institutionalized persons) in research; the nature of informed consent with incompetent persons; the possible coercion of parents to place their children in a research ward when no places were available in the general wards of the institution; and the possible alternative groups of patient subjects, other than institutionalized or vulnerable populations, that might have been used for these kinds of research studies.

From both studies it is possible to understand how ethical principles influence the selection of research subjects. Considering the principle of beneficence, we might think that the children in the Willowbrook Study were benefited by receiving a mild case of hepatitis, more personal attention, and residing in a better unit. Because they were benefited, the study was ethically justified. Yet we must ask if the principle of beneficence justifies experimentation when the benefit to be received is only realized because of the social condition in which the research subject finds himself. As had been pointed out by at least one ethicist, "any researcher encountering a group of subjects who will volunteer only because of their social condition has a moral duty to improve that condition rather than take advantage of it."(32) Thus, respect for the principle of beneficence would not have justified the choice of the children at Willowbrook for subjects in that study; neither would it have justified withholding penicillin from the syphilitic men in Macon County, Alabama.

Considering the principle of respect for persons, it is clear that the experiments did not treat the mentally retarded subject group—persons with diminished capacity to claim autonomy—as entitled to protection. There is also the serious question of whether subtle coercion was placed on parents of the Willowbrook children in order to obtain their consent. The waiting list for admittance to the institution was very long. Yet a retarded child could be admitted, without waiting, to the research unit. It is hard to see how this situation could be construed other than that of the undue influence on parental consent.

In the case of the Tuskegee study, respect for persons would not have allowed deception of the study participants nor would it have allowed the health of the community to be jeopardized by leaving a communicable disease untreated.

Consideration of the principle of justice also demonstrates that research subjects in both studies were not treated with equity. The Willowbrook children were a captive audience; therefore, they were vulnerable to exploitation by the researchers conducting the study. In the Tuskegee Study, the risks and benefits of the research were not distributed equally among the study participants.

How would the consideration of these principles affect studies conducted by nurses? In the ANA "Human Rights Guidelines," specific persons to whom the guidelines apply include "patients; outpatients; donors of organs, tissues, and services; informants; normal volunteers including students; and volunteers in groups with limited civil freedom," meaning prisoners, residents in institutions for the mentally ill or retarded, and persons subject to military discipline.(33) The "Human Rights Guidelines" note, all in these groups "tend to easily fall into the class of captive audience and population vulnerable to exploitation."(34) Thus, according to the standards of the nursing profession, equity in the selection of subjects (also non-discrimination against the sick, the prisoner, and the less fortunate), constitutes an important standard for research involving human subjects. Like informed consent, it is a necessary condition for ethically acceptable research.

I must point out, however, that the consequentalistic twist to nursing ethics again creeps in by this consideration of the selection of research subjects. The "Human Rights Guidelines" note that" . . . the choice of minors and groups with limited civil freedom as research subjects can be justified, in most instances, only if there are benefits that will accrue in the future to them or to others in similar situations or classes."(35) It seems as if the professional ethic supports a utilitarian notion of benefit to justify not protecting persons who have diminished capacity to claim autonomy. The important moral implications of this pronouncement are then sidestepped by the document's claim that government statutes and regulations are beginning to deal with standards for those lacking the capacity to give informed consent in research. This is certainly true as is attested by the "Final Regulations Amending Basic DHHS Policy for the Protection of Human Research Subjects." But the nursing profession, in order to meet accountability requirements (both personal and professional) expected by the public, needs to be clear about its own standards that guide research carried out to improve nursing practice.(36) How does the nurse investigator decide on future benefits and balance this against potential risks to research subjects and possible loss of autonomy?

Assessment of Risks and Benefits

This issue is one of the more difficult problems during the planning and writing of the research protocol. The researcher is expected to consider all possible consequences of the research study and is expected to balance any inherent risks to the research participant with proportionate benefits. To fail to do so is to undermine the moral justifications of the entire research study. First, the agents who are most likely to be subject to risk by the experiment must be identified. This could include the research subject, his family or even other groups in society. Second, the types of risk involved—physical, psychological or social—must be ascertained. Third, benefits to the various agents or others need to be identified and, if at all possible, quantified and balanced alongside the identified risks. In doing this kind of assessment, it is even helpful, and in some instances necessary, to include the viewpoints of others who are not institutionally connected to the research enterprise.(37) If a favorable benefit/risk ratio cannot be determined by this assessment process, the moral justification of the proposed research remains in question.

This is a potential conflict that has not gone unnoticed by the nursing profession. The concern for risk and benefits is worded very carefully in the "Human Rights Guidelines"

"... in situations in which the nature of the activities or research design exposes an individual to increased possibility of emotional, social, or physical injury, the degree of risk needs to be estimated and specified by the principle investigator or his designate. It is incumbent upon all practitioners to recognize that risk is potentially present in all situations when novel and untried procedures are involved and there is little if any data upon which to predict outcomes. The primary problem faced by the investigator or practitioner is prediction of the extent of risk to the individual in comparison to the potential clinical benefit to him and/or the humanitarian importance of the knowledge to be gained."(38)

It is interesting that this professional document refers to the "humanitarian importance of the knowledge to be gained" from research. The strong humanitarian concerns of nursing, the trust relationship shared by nurse and client, and the professional's primary commitment to client care and safety all dictate a strong duty of the nurse to protect research subjects from all possible harms encountered in a particular study. The principle of beneficence also requires researchers to engage in research for the benefit of the patient; in the case of research conducted by nurses, benefit for the patient is translated into the improvement of nursing practice. As the "Human Rights Guidelines" state, "By virtue of their calling, practitioners in the health professions seek to protect individuals under their care from arbitrary physical or mental suffering."(39)

The assessment of risks and benefits in research is thus an important issue in research and of particular moral significance to the nurse researcher. The principles of respect for persons, beneficence, and justice all require a very careful assessment of possible risks and benefits to client populations receiving nursing services in any form.

C. CONCLUSION

The practice of nursing and research to improve the practice of nursing are understandably influenced by the relevance of ethical principles and their priority in resolving ethical conflict. As the "Human Rights Guidelines" recognize, the nurse engaged in research values self-determination as a basic right of all persons, has a personal obligation to ensure and support self-determination of persons, and has a responsibility to safeguard the rights of others in research contexts. Thus, the principle of respect for persons has a very strong influence on nurse investigator behavior and modes of conduct throughout scientific inquiry.

But the principles of beneficence and justice also influence the nurse researcher. The nurse's primary commitment to client care and safety includes the duties to (1) provide maximum benefits to research subjects as well as other beneficiaries of the research study, (2) protect the patient from harm, and (3) make sure that clients are treated with equity. When these principles are consciously rendered their place of priority in research conducted by that nurse, then we can rightfully say that the practice of nursing is, indeed, improved through research.

ENDNOTES

1. The National Commission for the Protection of Human Subjects of Biomedical and Behavioral Research, The Belmont Report: Ethical Principles and Guidelines for the Protection of Human Subjects of Research; Washington: DEHW Publication NO. (OS) 78-0012, 1978, p. 2.
2. Ibid., p. 4.
3. Tom L. Beauchamp and James F. Childress, Principles of Biomedical Ethics; NY: Oxford, 1979, pp. 5–6.
4. Belmont, op. cit., p. 4.
5. Ibid., p. 5.
6. Ibid., p. 6.
7. Ibid., p. 7.
8. Ibid., p. 8; also, Beauchamp and Childress, op. cit., p. 168.
9. For a detailed analysis of seven major ethical issues in research, see LeRoy Walters, "Some Ethical Issues in Research Involving Human Subjects," Perspectives in Biology and Medicine (Winter 1977): 193–211.
10. Ibid., p. 195.
11. ANA, Human Rights Guidelines for Nurses in Clinical and Other Research; Kansas City, MO: ANA, 1975, p. 1.
12. Ibid., p. 6.
13. Ibid.
14. Ibid.
15. Belmont, op. cit., p. 10.
16. Ibid.
17. Federal Register 46 (26 Jan 81), 8366–8392.
18. ANA, op. cit., p. 7.
19. Belmont, op. cit., p. 11.
20. Beauchamp and Childress, op. cit., p. 65.
21. Ibid., p. 69.
22. Ibid.
23. Belmont, op. cit., p. 13.
24. ANA, op. cit., p. 8.
25. Ibid.

26. Beauchamp and Childress, op. cit., p. 80.

27. ANA, op. cit., p. 8.

28. For a good discussion of the ethical issues in this study, see Robert M. Veatch, Case Studies in Medical Ethics; Cambridge: Harvard, 1977, pp. 274–77.

29. Ibid., p. 275.

30. Allan M. Brandt, "Racism and Research: The Case of the Tuskegee Syphilis Study," HCR 8 (December 1978): 21.

31. Ibid.

32. Veatch, op. cit., p. 277.

33. ANA, op. cit., p. 5.

34. Ibid.

35. Ibid.

36. Sara T. Fry, "Accountability in Research: The Relationship of Scientific and Humanistic Values." ANS 4 (October 1981): 1–13.

37. Walters, op. cit., p. 200.

38. ANA. op. cit., p. 4.

39. Ibid.

CHAPTER 17

ETHICS OF NURSING RESEARCH BY THE CANADIAN NURSES' ASSOCIATION

[Research encompasses ethical concern for informed consent, confidentiality, and cost-benefit for the subject. The researcher needs to be competent and accountable. Participation must be compatible with nursing ethics. The setting needs appropriate resources and should be a place where the rights of all are protected.]

The Canadian Nurses' Association (Ottawa) published "Ethical Guidelines for Nursing Research Involving Human Subjects" (1983). It is based on the CNA Code of Ethics. These guidelines define nursing research "as a systematic controlled investigation involving human subjects directed to the advancement of nursing knowledge." There are three major divisions in the guidelines: (1) scientific merit; (2) human subject consent, confidentiality and protection; and (3) the setting. The latter includes the rights of others in the setting as well as a setting conducive to the research. That may include providing information to other staff who may have a right to withdraw from participation in the study. Subjects have a right to knowledge and understanding. The researcher has the responsibility to make sure the consent is freely given. This must be documented. The subject's confidentiality must be protected at all times. Either consent is given for the use of the material and/or anonymity must be preserved. Protection of the subject extends beyond the physical to the mental, emotional, and moral. Respect for persons means that in case of a conflict between the welfare of the person and the research, the person comes first. The first division asks whether the question is worth pursuing. Studies should be designed for reliability and validity and should involve optimum use of time and resources.

CHAPTER 18

HUMAN RIGHTS GUIDELINES FOR NURSES IN CLINICAL AND OTHER RESEARCH—ANA 1985

[The ANA is concerned with the rights of nurses and all persons involved in research. Human rights include freedom from injury and the right to privacy. Informed consent is a major source of assurance of these rights. Society, institutions, the professions, and individuals all carry responsibilities to support and protect human rights during research.]

In 1985, the American Nurses' Association Cabinet on Nursing Research issued the second edition of *Human Rights Guidelines for Nurses in Clincial and Other Research*. This important pamphlet contains background information on the development and need for guidelines when one involves human subjects in research activities, a summary of practical issues in the conduct of research and mechanisms for the protection of human subjects in research in addition to the Guidelines themselves. The focus of these human rights guidelines is Statement 7 of the ANA *Code for Nurses*, "The nurse participates in activities that contribute to the ongoing development of the profession's body of knowledge." The Guidelines are summarized below.

NURSING ACTIVITIES AND ETHICAL ISSUES

The generation and refinement of scientific knowledge in nursing has increasingly involved "nurses . . in clinical investigations that emphasize furthering knowledge rather than meeting the needs of patients. Ethical concerns about the potential violations of human rights become crucial when new and untried techniques and procedures are to be used or when the probable outcomes are unknown or doubtful."

The borderline between normal and experimental nursing and medi-

---

Reprinted with permission of the American Nurses' Association.

cal care has become blurred in recent times. Nurses have a right to protection from harm when involved in care with a research component just as clients or patients need to be protected from harm as participants in studies. Statements of employment should clearly indicate any special expectations about conditions, such as being part of double blind investigations, serving as data collectors, the option of not participating, etc. Work that entails risks must be noted along with information on recognizing the risk and action to counteract harmful effects.

PROTECTION OF HUMAN RIGHTS

Concerns for safeguarding the subject of human experimentation have been growing and have extended to such areas as death and dying, family planning, genetic engineering, manipulating behavior, and the allocation of resources. The human rights referred to in these guidelines include:

Right to freedom from intrinsic risk of injury

"In situations in which the nature of the activities or the research design exposes an individual to increased possibility of emotional, social or physical injury, the degree of risk must be estimated and specified by the principal investigator or designee." Full information that is clearly understood must be shared with prospective subjects prior to asking for consent to participate in activities that go beyond the normal or expected.

Right to privacy and dignity

Since human beings vary in their definition of what is considered an invasion of privacy, "all proposals, investigative instruments, protocols, and techniques to be used in particular activities and research methods must be specified and discussed with the prospective subject and with workers who are expected to participate in the activity as subjects, data collectors, or both."

Right to anonymity

"Safeguards must be developed so that no unanticipated physical, psychological, or social disadvantage accrues to subjects either during the study or as a result of the dissemination of findings. . . . Special mechanisms for safeguarding confidentiality and protecting the identity of a subject must be developed if the information is not to remain always under the control of the investigator."

SUBJECTS

The patient-nurse relationship involves trust as recognized by professional codes of ethics. In research, the investigator assumes special obligations for safeguarding the subject with special sensitivity to captive and vulnerable populations. "The choice of minors and groups with limited civil freedom as research subjects can be justified in most instances only if benefits will accrue in the future to them or to others in similar situations or classes."

SOCIETY'S OBLIGATIONS AND THE PUBLIC GOOD

"In a democratic society, the rights of individuals are of necessity counterbalanced by actions and activities designed for the common good of the collective public. . . . Advancement of knowledge about health and health-promoting practices is of value to society as a whole." Nurses must continue the advance of knowledge and support qualified nurse-scientists as they carry out the pursuit of knowledge through research.

SECTION VII
THE TEACHING OF ETHICS

CHAPTER 19

INTEGRATING ETHICS CONTENT INTO THE NURSING CURRICULA

Joyce E. Thompson and Henry O. Thompson

[Ethics education for nurses is mandatory, yet not all nursing schools provide ethics education in an organized manner. This essay explores, and offers suggestions on, the ethics content needed across the three levels of nursing programs, the sequencing of that content, how and who should teach it, and how ethics can be evaluated.]

Nurses are expected to practice in an ethical manner. It has been suggested that to be professional is to be ethical and to be unethical is to be unprofessional. The very concept of profession carries with it something far more than the job or employment part of life. It is, in fact, a way of life. A nursing education, then, is not just a technical training program to teach people how to run machinery or make a bed. It is concerned with the entire profession of nursing, including its ethical standards. These, in turn, reflect the whole of society and, indeed, humanity.

The codes of ethics for professional nursing are one symbol of the importance of ethical standards in nursing.(1) In turn, they reinforce the professional concept that ethics is a crucial part of nursing. As such, it *should* be taught. Many suggest that ethics is taught whether anyone likes it or not, or, perhaps one could say it is "caught" by students who learn from the behaviors modeled by teachers and nursing colleagues. This process will not stop by officially including ethics in the curriculum. However, including ethics in the nursing curriculum is a more professional way of teaching it rather than leaving such a crucial aspect of nursing to "chance". Teaching ethics makes such content specific and public, and therefore open to critical examination and reflection.

Integrating ethics into the nursing curricula has engendered much discussion during the past decade.(2) There are several issues involved in ethics teaching. What ethics content is needed in nursing? When should it be taught? How should it be taught? Who should teach it? How can it be evaluated? The purpose of this essay is to consider each of these questions related to integrating and teaching ethics across the nursing curricula. Our concern is teachers and those with a commitment to improve the ethical dimensions of nursing.(3)

BACKGROUND MATERIAL

There are three assumptions inherent in this discussion. First, ethics is vital to any health-related profession. To be a professional requires ethical behavior. To practice ethically requires knowledge of what it means to be ethical. With this commitment, time and effort will be given to the teaching of ethics in the professional schools.

The second assumption is that ethics, morality, and values can be taught and learned. There is an old debate, "Are we good by nature or can we be taught to be good?" One answer is "both." Education is the primary variable in the natural law theories of Lawrence Kohlberg and his concept of moral development.(4) Some value theorists say we internalize most of our primary values and moral positions by the age of ten.(5) However, values can be changed through awareness. With or without change, we can understand our own values and those of others.

The third assumption is that ethical concerns and moral decisions are a daily part of nursing.(6) One could say there is an ethical dimension to every decision made in nursing practice, as well as in every interaction between human beings—whether it be client/nurse, student/teacher, nurse/physician, or nurse/community.(7) In addition to the personal dimension, ethical nursing practice is an essential part of the social contract of professionals.(8) Nurses have certain moral obligations and duties to society as well as rights and privileges accorded by society as a direct result of being a nurse.

Formal preparation for ethical decision making, however, has lagged behind our recognition of the need. It may be that most nursing educators and practitioners believe that their students already know the right thing to do (intuitionism). Or perhaps they have not thought about the ethical dimensions of professional nursing enough to accord them a place in the nursing curriculum. Another reason has been shared in various consultations and conversations on this topic throughout the nation. Some faculty see themselves as having limited expertise in defining and teaching ethics. The nurse faculty may be threatened by the philosophical and religious foundations of ethics. They do not have resources for teaching ethics, so no one does it (officially). One way we deal with threatening content as teachers is to avoid it.

However, we teach by precept and example. Ethics can be learned. We need to know how and what to teach. That brings us to specific ethics content that should be taught, when it should be taught (organization/ framework), how and by whom. As with any reasoned approach to learning and professional practice, the evaluation of what has been learned from teaching and student application of knowledge will be the final area for discussion. We begin with the definition of ethics content.

DEFINITION OF ETHICS CONTENT

Nursing ethics is generally described as "normative" ethics, the category of ethical inquiry which tells people how they *should* act or what they *should* do in a given situation. Normative or prescriptive ethics involves both theory and application. Exploration of how nurses reason morally and make ethical decisions also requires examination of values and moral development. These are examples of "descriptive" ethics— what is or exists within the individual at a given point in time. Both aspects of ethics education are required, as nurses are persons who are learning what they *should* do and how it might differ from what they *would* do without prior reflection.

Definitions

Definition of common terms used in discussing morals and ethics are an important beginning. There is some debate among ethicists and philosophers on the definitions of ethics, morals, metaethics, values, and beliefs. However, it is important to present a glossary that is clear and useful to both teachers and students. Ethics may involve a new vocabulary for both. Clarity in meaning will help diminish the threat to learning ethics.

We have found it helpful to distinguish morals as the "shoulds and oughts of professional practice" and ethics as the "reasons why." A learner's response or action in a given situation is followed by an ethical, "Why?" This reinforces the importance of making a decision as well as understanding the reasoning used for it. In the sense of "should" and "why", the ANA *Code for Nurses*(9) eleven precepts are moral prescriptions and the Interpretive Statements explain the ethical justification for each.

One can also begin with definitions of values, beliefs, attitudes, and values clarification. A comparison of the nursing process with the moral reasoning process is helpful as well. Thus, one begins with the familiar (nursing process) and builds on the student's prior learning. The glossary may be provided or developed with the learners as ethics education progresses. A good road map in easily understood language can be a very helpful tool in the teaching of ethics.

Theory

The descriptive theories of how people develop morally are important building blocks for discussion of ethical nursing practice.(10) This content is basic to the understanding of human nature and what it means to be a moral agent. Nurses are moral agents, as are other health professionals.(11) Nurses need to understand and integrate the concept of being a moral agent as they learn to be a nurse.

Values clarification is an important part of ethics education in nursing.(12) Nurses need to explore the values they brought with them to nursing as well as the values inherent in the profession.(13) This includes analysis of the values and ethical dimensions of professional documents such as the ANA *Code for Nurses, Standards of Nursing Practice,* and the ANA *Social Policy Statement.*(14) Students need to know if their personal and professional values are congruent, or divergent, or need changing, and which values are appropriate and applicable to their professional role.

The theory base for nursing ethics includes the major philosophical systems of bioethics. These are utilitarianism, deontology, and natural law, though the latter may be viewed as a combination of both the former.(15) The deontological system of ethics consists of ethical principles and moral rules. An important part of the theory is definition and discussion of these principles with particular emphasis on those affecting nursing, including research. Examples are truthtelling, respect for the personhood (human dignity) of all people, the Golden Rule, autonomy and self-determination of clients and professionals, beneficence (doing good) and nonmaleficence (at least do no harm), informed consent and client participation in decisions about their care, and just allocation of scarce resources.(16) The ethical obligations, duties, and rights of nurses as professionals are important as well.(17)

APPLICATION OF ETHICS THEORY

Applied ethics in nursing includes how to reason morally, how to identify the ethical dimensions of nursing practice, and how to make ethical decisions in practice. Case studies provide the building blocks.

Moral reasoning is vital. It can be compared to the nursing process with emphasis on identifying and critically analyzing the ethical dimensions of nursing. Moral reasoning can be learned (understood) and modeled, and frequent use results in successful integration into the learner's professional practice. Nurses are involved in making decisions for and about patients and clients. A reasoned approach provides a basis for that decision making.(18)

Applied ethics includes how to decide whether to begin resuscitation on a 500-gram infant born 20 weeks early to a woman who had no prenatal care or what to do when the parents of a severely ill and dying neonate ask for use of all technology possible. Other ethical dilemmas include how to allocate nursing time and expertise to individual patients when there is a shortage of nurses or what to do if you are asked to care for a very ill patient and you do not know how to provide that care. When to call a code for a person with terminal cancer or what to do if you disagree with a "do not resuscitate" order for a given patient, highlight some of the difficult ethical decisions required at the end of life. Issues concerning the allocation of resources, truthtelling, quality of life, and euthanasia are but a few of those encountered daily in the nurse's life.(19)

The historical, philosophical, and current social ethics related to these issues required discussion to understand why we do what we do today. This understanding may also help us to critically evaluate whether what is currently being done is appropriate for our time and society. History is vital lest we repeat the mistakes of the past as we search for the right answers in today's complex and confusing society as well as in that microcosm of society—the health and illness care system.

Part of that complexity is biomedical technology.(20) The interface of ethics and law is another content issue.(21) Too often the nurse defers to the legal dimensions for fear of reprisal. Both ethics and legalities need consideration. Smith and Davis.(22) have pointed out that there are actions we take in nursing practice which are both ethical and legal, others which are legal but unethical, and still others which are ethical but illegal.

In summary, the theoretical and applied content in ethics teaching includes definitions, philosophical systems of ethics, moral development, values and valuing, moral reasoning and ethical decision making, ethical issues in the life cycle, and the interface of ethics, law, and biomedical technology. This content is geared toward defining what it means to be a professional nurse, one who knows and practices in an ethical manner.

GOALS OF ETHICS EDUCATION

Callahan and others(23) have offered several goals for teaching ethics to professionals. They can be summarized as follows:

1. **Stimulate the moral imagination** so the student is helped to recognize his/her own values and understand there *is* a moral point of view in life, although hidden at times. Teachers need to facilitate the learner's ability to differentiate what "feels" right or good from what "is" right or good.

2. **Recognize ethical issues** including the learner's ability to identify the moral or ethical dimensions of nursing practice, the existence of a moral dilemma, and how ethical theory can be applied to the situation in order to make an ethical decision for action.

3. **Elicit a sense of moral obligation.** Ethical thinking requires us to act in the light of what we/profession/society perceive to be right and good. Ethical analysis cannot be separated from a sense of moral obligation to do the best we can (in contrast to doing what can be argued best). Individuals have some freedom to make moral choices in life, but they are also responsible for the choices they make.

4. **Develop analytical skills.** Consistency and clarity are minimal goals in the analysis of ethical propositions and in their justification, tempered with caring and compassion.[24] We need to articulate our moral positions and ethical reasoning if we expect them to be heard and respected.

5. **Tolerate and reduce disagreements and ambiguity.** Moral dilemmas should force a grappling with the nature of the moral life itself. This can be a frustrating part of ethics learning as nurses generally have not been taught to reason philosophically or live with uncertainties of action. The teacher's role is to help the learners tolerate disagreement and ambiguity, to respect others, and to disagree without personal attack as they learn what it means to be moral agents in society.

CONCEPTUAL FRAMEWORK

The conceptual framework for nursing ethics may be described as the ethics of caring. There are three vital components to it: compassion, competence, and convenant fidelity. Each of these components can be woven throughout the teaching of ethics theory and its application to the practice of nursing.(25)

TEACHING ETHICS CONTENT TO ADULTS

Teaching should be in accord with principles of learning applied to how adults learn, the type of knowledge to be taught, and the topic. Teaching methods helpful in other disciplines may be helpful in teaching ethics. These include lecture/discussion, group discussion, simulation exercises, values clarification, case analysis, self-study, team presentations, audiovisuals, ethics rounds, and individual counseling sessions. Several authors describe the advantages and disadvantages of these methods for ethics teaching.(26)

Those persons teaching ethics, morals, and values need to recognize what the learner brings to the teaching situation. New concepts can create affective dissonance in learners so that they are motivated to explore their personal value sets, examine alternatives, and then move on to choose new values or keep the former which fit their developing professional role in nursing.(27) The guiding principle for integrating ethics content has been that a sound theoretical foundation in ethics is a must for ethical reasoning.(28)

The focus of the present essay is the selection of specific teaching methods based on the content in ethics being taught. We begin with a review of how adults learn and the use of this theory in selecting one's teaching methods for ethics.

How Adults Learn

Malcolm Knowles is a proponent of andragogy, the science of teaching adults. He believes that adults learn differently than children. Adult educational efforts should be designed differently than pedagogy. There are several assumptions in his theory. Adult learners are self-directing, capable of taking responsibility for their own learning. Educators need to actively involve the adult learner in setting goals for the educational experience, facilitating the learner's efforts to learn by discovery, critical thinking, and application of theory in practice. In ethics teaching, this means that learners need to be encouraged and supported as they grapple with ethical theories and their application to nursing practice. It is important to encourage the learners to spend more time on the process of moral reasoning than on working toward consensus for action. This is especially true in the early stages.

Some students complain that studying ethics won't make them a better nurse like studying disease prevention and learning basic nursing skills. This thought is most common in the early stages of ethics study and more often than not, comes from one who has yet to practice nursing. It may also be a reflection of a lack of commitment by the faculty or nursing program to the value of ethics education. If the teachers of ethics are the only ones committed to ethics education, the rest of the faculty and school can undermine ethics learning by their refusal to integrate a discussion of ethics in every nursing course. Students carry more than one course at a time, and can quickly spot the inconsistencies in the curriculum as evidenced in the value-laden teaching of each faculty member.

The second assumption in the andragogical method is that adults enter into educational activities with both a greater volume and a different quality of experience than children. Adults are often the richest resources for one another. This suggests that group discussion, simulation exercises in values clarification, and problem-solving projects that encourage and support the adults' exploration of their personal experiences and beliefs about ethics and learning from other people's varying values and beliefs might work best in ethics education.

The assumption about the experiential background of adult learners is of interest in the sequencing of ethics content, noted in the following section. Freshman or sophomore nursing students bring a personal life history to ethics education, but may have minimal life experience in the day-to-day nursing world. Graduate nursing students have a more extensive professional nursing base but this can cause a narrowing of their ethical vision. The "reality" of nursing may limit their list of alternative nursing actions based on ethical reasoning. Having a mix of age and educational levels in the same ethics classroom can be frustrating, but highly challenging and motivating for all participants as they struggle to understand each other and how their ethical or moral stances came to be.

The third assumption of the andragogical model is that adults become ready to learn (a necessary condition for all learning) when they experience a need to know or do something. This may be in order to perform more effectively in some aspect of their lives. Teachers can also induce readiness to learn. They can expose the learners to more effective role models. Students can be engaged in discussion that triggers their value positions and exposes conflicts with these positions. The teacher can provide diagnostic experiences in which they can assess the gaps between where they are now and where they want and need to be as professional nurses.

The fourth assumption about adult learners is that they enter an educational activity with a life-centered, task-centered, or problem-centered orientation. For the most part, adults learn in order to be able to perform a task, solve a problem, or live in a more satisfying way. One implication of this assumption is the importance of designing learning experiences around real life or "actual" nursing situations rather than using "artificial" cases.

The final assumption is about the adult's motivation to learn. The andragogical model assumes that the more potent motivators of adults are internal—self-esteem, recognition, better quality of life, greater self-confidence, and self-actualization. Our educational systems often socialize learners to the docile acceptance of the pearls of wisdom of the teacher. External motivators such as rewards for a correct answer are part of the system. These can be changed as the learner recognizes that ethical nursing practice is internally motivated. How we perform when no one else is watching is a more important indicator of our "ethicalness" than what we do when we know someone is watching. This statement is based on the assumption that the teacher accepts this fact about ethics and encourages discussion.

TEACHING METHODS BY LEVEL OF STUDENT AND CONTENT AREA

Use of lectures and discussion during the introductory phases of ethics theory is one way to assist the learner in attaining a solid theory base in ethics. Ethics theory can also be learned through use of selected audiovisuals, such as Morris Massey's video tapes on values. Exercises in values clarification are also important teaching tools. They increase learner participation as well as respectful discourse.

As one proceeds to applied ethics content, teaching methods can change to include case study and analysis. Cases can be found in the literature or drawn from personal experience—both the teacher's and the students'.

The selection of the cases for analysis is important. Selection for the purpose at hand can expedite learning. Cases which highlight values are useful in values clarification. These may take the form of adding blank parentheses behind each value variable (sex, age, prognosis, religious belief, family wishes, client wishes) to be highlighted during discussion of an actual case. Individuals can work alone or within a small group with the directions to read and study the case. Priorities can be assigned to the parenthetical variables. These reflect the importance each variable carries with the learners as they make a decision for action in the situation. Number 1 usually indicates the highest priority and higher numbers a lower priority. Once the individual or group has completed their prioritizing, group discussion can then focus on why these variables were placed as they were in the hierarchy of value. This discussion can also highlight the varying value systems of the participants, with careful attention to maintaining the confidentiality of those who desire it.

Later stages of application need cases that emphasize moral reasoning. The actual actions taken in the situation may not be known. It is the reasoning process that is important. Thompson and Thompson, *Bioethical Decision Making for Nurses* (1985), presents a ten-step decision model based on moral reasoning which requires a critical and orderly analysis of clinical or research situations.

Cases with known outcomes can be used for a different assignment, including film and videotapes with an ethics theme. Students are asked to evaluate decisions and actions in terms of ethical theory, with reasons for and against the action. Learners can also be asked for alternative actions that might have been considered in the situation, and thus be encouraged to expand their own thinking on alternatives in similar clinical situations. Retrospective analysis of cases also reflect a reality in nursing practice. In an emergency, there is insufficient time to thoroughly reason through the situation and investigate alternative actions that are both possible and justifiable prior to taking action. A note of caution is in order, however. If retrospective review is the only case analysis used in teaching, this may be the approach used most often in the learner's nursing practice (modeling). Critical thinking *prior* to making ethical decisions should be done whenever possible. Therefore, a majority of the case studies used for teaching should require pre-decision reasoning.

Ethics rounds and conferences on ethical issues are common teaching methodologies used in continuing education programs. They can also be useful as part of the standard curricula. These teaching methods usually have a case or an issue focus, and limit the amount of information which can be shared about ethics. Time available for such ethics rounds is usually limited, so the teacher must assume an ethics theory base among learners or plan a brief introduction. Fortunately, ethics rounds often are scheduled on a continuing basis, so ethics content can be expanded over time, providing the same learners avail themselves of each session.

Undergraduate Content

One approach is to begin with a freshman-sophomore level theory course that provides a base on which other nursing courses can build in applying ethics. Within the beginning theory course, the approach varies according to the background of the students. Lecture complimented by discussion and liberal use of audiovisual aids are appropriate to the presentation of ethics theory. Ordinarily, one would expect nursing experience to be at a minimum. This may not be the case with second career students, RNs seeking a baccalaureate, or students who choose a nursing career after working in first aid or hospitals. But one can count on life experience as background regardless of the amount of nursing experience.

A general introduction to ethics can use life experiences ranging from student problems like cheating, the fairness of college selection policies, interpersonal relations ranging from child-parent to woman-man, job experiences that may involve honest work for honest pay or integrity in business or politics. General situations, or shared experiences from faculty and students can be discussed in terms of ethics theories. The educational concept here is the old one of moving from the familiar to the less familiar, or from the known to the unknown. Experience with other kinds of theory such as geometry have also proven helpful. Some people can remember their childhood well enough and some are old enough to have children of their own. Some can remember asking, "Why?"—the philosophical question raised in relation to the moral standard. They may also remember the parental metaethic, "Because I said so, that's why!" as the ultimate axiom of appeal. Careful analogies can facilitate understanding of the ethical "why?".

Opportunities for moral development may appear if an ethics theory differs from the learner"s personal moral standards. Discussion can help understanding, which may show the adequacy of the earlier standard while exploring the pluralistic nature of society. Or, it may show the inadequacy of the earlier, and indicate directions of change, as when self-centered people move to a social orientation, from Kohlberg's Level I to Level II.(29)

At the junior and senior levels of nursing, opportunities for application of ethics theory are many. A beginning focus on ethical principles and issues, such as client autonomy and self-determination in a medical/surgical setting, or adolescent sexuality and contraception in a family planning setting, can be introduced within each clinical nursing course. Senior leadership courses are excellent forums for discussion of what it means to be a professional, to be ethical. A question that usually results in much discussion is, "At what time in your basic nursing education should you be held accountable for professional nursing behaviors?" The reader will have many of his/her own professional questions which will encourage discussion and exploration of professional ethics and values.

Master's Level

Ethics theory can be applied more directly to nursing experience when students have such experience. Graduate students are more likely to have work experience in nursing. They still need the theory if they do not already have it. A short introduction provides a review of ethics theory for those who have had formal study already, and directed reading can assist those without earlier study to build on the class introduction. The introduction also provides common ground for the class. Both moral philosophers and moral theologians frequently emphasize different aspects of ethics theory, so the mere fact of prior study does not ensure common knowledge. The differences can add to the discussion and be a rich resource for further growth and development.

In the upper classes and graduate school, case studies provide a practical approach that some nurses appreciate. Dividing a class into small groups of 5 to 10 people allows maximum participation. Cases provide opportunities to discuss real issues in the calm of the classroom without the pressures of immediate decision making often required in the work setting. As noted earlier, without a theoretical framework, discussion can be merely "shooting the breeze." The ethical "Why?" is a significant portion of the analysis of the case.

Stating one's position could be helpful as an indication of one's values. Values clarification can, in turn, help both speaker and group to understand the background of the position and its degree of adequacy. There is a reminder here that we need to try to understand the values and the motivations of others as well as ourselves because this knowledge is very important in working with patients, with health care colleagues, or simply with other human beings. But we may have more opportunity to clarify our own values when, or if, we can be genuinely honest with ourselves. This is a major part of the interaction we have with others. Creating a climate of mutual respect and trust in the classroom is imperative when one expects honest sharing of values and moral positions.(30)

Personal values clarification is also appropriate in relation to a theory of moral development such as Kohlberg's. When people with different values are willing to share those, it is not unusual to find persons at different stages or levels of moral development. In Kohlberg's work, people do not understand two stages or more above their own. They do understand the next stage and exposure to it can help them develop further. This suggests another value for group discussion of ethics, including analysis of cases. It helps people grow in their own moral development.(31)

Doctoral Level

As noted earlier, the doctoral student interested in ethics is probably in the best position to add to our current knowledge base in ethics, particularly nursing ethics. This presumes a theory base in bioethics and requires a broad knowledge and understanding of ethics, moral development as well as research methodologies appropriate to ethics exploration. Many doctoral studies have contributed to our understanding of moral development and how nurses make ethical decisions, but much more knowledge is needed.(32) Teaching methodology supports self-study and promotes creative thinking in a mentor relationship.

In summary, theory is a prerequisite to applied ethics. You cannot apply theory if you do not know it. The philosophical and religious basis of this theory is often taught by lectures, followed by group discussion and sharing. This allows the lecturer with knowledge of philosophical and theological ethics to synthesize material and present it in a manner that is understandable and non-threatening to the learner. Group discussion is essential for assessing the level of understanding of ethics theory. Learners, however, may get impatient because they want the application made clear, right now! The temptation is to use case studies before a solid theory foundation is laid. The theory provides a basis for analyzing the cases. Without the theory, discussion may be simply a trading of opinions without understanding. Without the reality of nursing practice, theory stands in danger of being mere speculation. The interaction of theory and reality can strengthen both. Short-term excitement may be traded for the long-term gain of better decision making with a fuller background in ethics theory.

WHO SHOULD TEACH ETHICS

In many ways, the response to this question is quite obvious. The persons who should teach ethics in nursing are those qualified to do so. Qualifications include experience in education, so that they can adapt teaching methods to the content and level of the learners. They should have expertise in ethics as well as in nursing and the ability to share that expertise in a meaningful and understanding manner. They should be individuals who create a trusting learning environment where values, beliefs, and moral positions can be shared without reprisal or condemnation.

Sometimes such individuals are not available. Some schools use a team teaching approach. A nurse joins with a philosopher, clergy and/or ethicist with an interest/awareness in nursing. This joint effort has the advantages of introducing a non-nursing perspective into clinical decision-making and a non-philosophical perspective into discussions of ethics theory. This combination can help the philosophers avoid spending all of their time in theoretical clouds and the nurses avoid spending all their time in reality shock.

All nurse educators have a role in teaching applied ethics. They may need additional knowledge to increase their understanding and application of ethics theory to clinical practice. The ethical dimensions of professional nursing require all nurses to be knowledgeable in ethics.

EVALUATION OF ETHICS LEARNING

The theory portion of ethics content can be tested in written essays or objective tests like any other theory. Term papers can be assigned to explore one or two facets and this theory. The same techniques may be appropriate for values clarification. The concern here is to check understanding, rather than memorization of facts or theories, although the theory of values clarification itself is significant. Cases studies are appropriate to test skills of analysis. These may be selected in terms of whether it is a pre-decision analysis coming to a decision or retroactive analysis of the decisions already made, both demonstrating the reasoning process itself. In addition to cognitive understanding and articulation, affective objectives need not be overlooked. The relationship between Kohlberg's reasoning stages of moral development and the affective domain is still being debated.(33) But compassion, caring, sensitivity, commitment, feelings about the importance of ethics can be recognized even when, or if, they cannot be quantitatively measured. Faculty often claim objectivity as the desideratum but qualitative judgments are also part of the evaluation.(34)

In the clinical setting, the learner's approach to client care, co-workers and faculty can be evaluated in terms of the ethical mandates of nursing. Participation in class discussions is also an important tool for evaluating the progress of learners in integrating ethics content in their thinking and practice.

SUMMARY

We have offered suggestions on what ethics content should be taught in nursing curricula, how, when and who should teach it, and how it can be evaluated. If we expect nurses to assume responsibility for practicing in an ethical manner, we cannot remain in a merely consultant role, called in to pronounce judgment on the rights and wrongs of a thorny moral dilemma. Ethical nursing practice is a responsibility of every nurse, and ethics can be learned. Ethics is also a matter of individuals choosing morally justifiable actions and accepting responsibility for them as a member of society as well as a practitioner in the profession of nursing. We can no longer ignore the equation of ethics and nursing. Ethics education for nurses is mandatory, not elective.

ENDNOTES

1. American Nurses Association, *Code for Nurses with Interpretive Statements,* Kansas City, MO: The Association, 1985. See also the ICN Code of Ethics in Barbara L. Tate, *The Nurse's Dilemma: Ethical Considerations in Nursing Practice.* Geneva: ICN, 1977.

2. Mila A. Aroskar, "Ethics in the Nursing Curriculum," NO 25, No. 4 (1977), 260–264. Id., "Anatomy of an Ethical Dilemma," (in this volume). Myra E. Levine, "Nursing Ethics and the Ethical Nurse," (in this volume). Margaret O. Steinfels, "Ethics, Education and Nursing Practice," HCR 7 (1977), 20–21. Joyce E. Thompson and Henry O. Thompson, "Teaching Ethics to Nurse-Midwives," JNM 23, No. 2 (1978), 31–35. Id., "Ethical Decision Making in Nursing," MCN 6, No. 1 (1981), 21–23, 60. Rita J. Payton, "Bioethical Program for Baccalaureate Nursing Students," *ANA Publication (G-145),* 1980, pp. 53–65. A.T. Stanley, "Ethics in Nursing Practice and Education: Curriculum Considerations," ibid., pp. 39–52. S. Andrews & S.A. Hutchinson, "Teaching Nursing Ethics: A Practical Approach," JNE 20, No. 1 (1981), 6–11. Patricia A. Munhall, "Moral Development: A Prerequisite," JNE 21, No. 6 (1982), 11–15. Mila A. Aroskar and Robert M. Veatch, "Ethics Teaching in Nursing Schools," HCR 7 (1977), 24–26.

3. Thompson and Thompson, "Should Nurses Study Ethics?" (In this volume). Lucie Young Kelly, *Dimensions of Professional Nursing,* 3rd ed; NY: Macmillan, 1981, Ch 13, "Professional Ethics and Accountability." Mila A. Aroskar, "Are Nurses' Mind Sets Compatible with Ethical Practice?" TCN 4, No. 1 (1982), 22–32.

4. Lawrence Kohlberg, *Essays on Moral Development.* Vol. 1 (1981) *The Philosophy of Moral Development;* Vol. 2. (1984) *The Psychology of Moral Development;* NY: Harper & Row.

5. Morris Massey, "What you are is . . ." [video]; Boulder, CO: Massey

Associates, 1980. Erik Erikson, *Childhood and Society;* NY: Norton, 1950. Abraham Maslow, *New Knowledge in Human Values;* NY: Harper & Row, 1959. Jean Piaget, *The Moral Development of the Child;* NY: Free Press, 1965 (original 1932). Louis E. Raths, Merrill Harmin and Sidney B. Simon, *Values and Teaching,* 2nd ed; Columbus: Merrill, 1978. Diane B. Uustal provides a suscinct review of value theory in her *Values and Ethics in Nursing: From Theory to Practice;* East Greenwich, RI: Educational Resources in Nursing and Wholistic Health, 1985, pp. 87–104.

6. Thompson and Thompson, *Ethics and Nursing;* NY: Macmillan, 1981, ch. 2 [cited hereafter as TTE]. Anne J. Davis and Mila A. Aroskar, *Ethical Dilemmas and Nursing Practice,* 2nd ed; Norwalk, CT: Appleton-Century-Crofts, 1983. Leah Curtin and M. Josephine Flaherty, *Nursing Ethics: Theories and Pragmatics;* Bowie, MD: Brady, 1982.

7. Jacques Barzun, "The Professions Under Siege," *Harper's Magazine* 257 (1978), 61–68. Thompson and Thompson, *Bioethical Decision Making for Nurses;* Norwalk: A-C-C, 1985 [cited hereafter as TTB].

8. Curtin & Flaherty, op. cit., pp. 67–78.

9. *Code for Nurses,* op. cit.

10. Jean Piaget and Barbara Inhelder, *The Psychology of the Child;* NY: Basic, 1969. Kohlberg, op. cit.

11. TTB-49-73.

12. Shirley M. Steele & Vera M. Harmon, *Values Clarification in Nursing,* 2nd ed; Norwalk: Appleton-Century-Crofts, 1983. Uustal, op. cit. Id., *Values and Ethics: Considerations in Nursing Practice;* Deerfield, MA: Uustal, 1978.

13. TTB-77-83, 129–134. Margot J. Fromer, "Solving Ethical Dilemmas in Nursing Practice," TCN 4, No. 1 (1982), 15–21. E. Crowder, "Manners, Morals and Nurses: An Historical Overview of Nursing Ethics," *Texas Reports on Biology and Medicine* 32, No. 1 (1974). 173–80. *Perspectives on the Code for Nurses;* Kansas City, MO: ANA, 1976.

14. Documents published by the ANA.

15. Tom L. Beauchamp & James F. Childress, *Principles of Biomedical Ethics,* 2nd ed; NY: Oxford, 1983. TTB-72-43. Kurt Baier, "Ethics. IV. Teleological Theories," EB 1:417–421. Id., "Ethics III: Deontological Theories," EB 1:413–417.

16. Code for Nurses, op. cit. Steele & Harmon, op. cit. TTB-83.

17. Sharon J. Smith and Anne J. Davis, "Ethical Dilemmas: Conflicts Among Rights, Duties, Obligations," this volume.

18. TTB-89-101. D. F. Allen & Marsha D. Fowler, "Cognitive Moral Development Theory and Moral Decisions in Health Care," *Law, Medicine & Health Care* 10 (1982), 19–23. Andrew J. Jameton, "The Nurse: When Roles Conflict," HCR 7 (1977), 22–23. Theresa Stanley, "Nursing," EB 3:1138–1146. Curtin & Flaherty, op. cit., pp. 59–63. Shakte Ketefian, "Education for Ethical Decision Making," *NLN Publication (15–2154);* 1986, pp. 135–146. E.O. Bridston, "An Educational Strategy for Enhancement of Moral-Ethical Decision Making," TCN 4, No. 1 (1982), 57–65.

19. TTE. Elsie L. Bandman & Bertram Bandman, *Nursing Ethics in the Life Span;* Norwalk, CT: Appleton-Century-Crofts, 1985.

20. Gina Corea, *The Mother Machine: Reproductive Technologies from Artificial Insemination to Artificial Wombs;* NY: Harper & Row, 1985. Jeffrey Lyons, *Playing God in the Nursery;* NY: Norton, 1985. Helen B. Holmes, Betty Hoskins and Michael Gross, eds., *The Custom Made Child?;* Clifton, NJ: Humana, 1980. D.N. Walton, *Ethics of Withdrawal of Life Support Systems;* Westport, CT: Greenwood, 1983.

21. K.M. Fenner, *Ethics and Law in Nursing: Professional Perspectives;* NY: Van Nostrand, 1980. Eugene I. Pavlon, *Human Rights and Health Care Law;* NY: AJN, 1980. A.J. Rosoff, *Informed Consent: A Guide for Health Care Providers;* Rockville, MD: Aspen, 1981.

22. Smith & Davis, op. cit.

23. Danial Callahan & Sisela Bok, *Ethics Teaching in Higher Education;* NY: Plenum, 1980. Catherine P. Murphy, "The Moral Situation in Nursing," in *Bioethics and Human Rights* ed. Bandman & Bandman; Boston: Little, Brown, 1978. Raths, Harmin & Simon, op. cit.

24. B.A. Carper, "The Ethics of Caring," ANS 1, No. 3 (1979), 11. Myra E. Levine, op. cit. Aroskar, Anatomy, op. cit. Carol Gilligan, *In a Different Voice;* Cambridge: Harvard, 1982.

25. Thompson & Thompson, "The Ethic of Caring: A Guide for Health Professionals," forthcoming.

26. Bridston, op. cit. C. Gilbert, "The What and How of Ethics Education," TCN 4, No. 1 (1982), 49–56. Marvin W. Berkowitz, "The Role of Discussion in Ethics Training," TCN 4, No. 1 (1982), 33–48. Fromer, op. cit. Id., "Teaching Ethics by Case Analysis," NO 28, No. 10 (1980), 604–609. Payton, op. cit. K.O. Vito, "Moral Development Considerations in Nursing Curricula," JNE 22, No. 3 (1983), 108–113. R. Feather, "Hypothetical Dilemmas—A Teaching Strategy for Moral Development," JNE 24, No. 7 (1985), 298–301. Robert M. Veatch, *Case Studies in Medical Ethics;* Cambridge: Harvard, 1977. Minerva L. Applegate & Nina M. Entrekin, *Teaching Ethics in Nursing: A Handbook for the Use of the Case-Study Method Approach;* NY: NLN, 1984, pp. i–iv, 1–81. Patricia L. Munhall, "Methodologic Fallacies: A Critical Self-Appraisal," ANS 5, No. 4 (1983), 41–49. *Ethics References for Nurses;* Kansas City, MO: ANA, 1982. T.K. McElhinney, ed., *Human Values Teaching Programs for Health Professionals;* Ardmore, PA: Whitmore, 1981.

27. Malcolm S. Knowles, *The Modern Practice of Adult Education,* rev; San Francisco: Jossey-Bass, 1980. Knowles, et al., *Andragogy in Action;* San Francisco: Jossey-Bass, 1984.

28. TTB-79-81. Steele & Harmon, op. cit., p. 7. Howard Brody, *Ethical Decisions in Medicine;* Boston: Little, Brown, 1976. S.B. Simon & J. Clark, *Beginning Values Clarification;* San Diego: Pennant, 1975. A.M. Woodruff, "Becoming a Nurse: The Ethical Perspective," *International Journal of Nursing Studies* 22, No. 4 (1985), 295–302.

29. Kohlberg, op. cit.

30. TTB-78.

31. Kohlberg, op. cit. Munhall, op. cit. James Rest, "The Cognitive Developmental Approach to Morality: The State of the Art," *Counseling and Values* 18, No. 2 (1974), 64–78. See also Rest, *Development in Judging Moral Issues;* Minneapolis: University of Minnesota, 1979. Id., *Moral Development: Advances in Research and Theory;* NY: Praeger, 1986.

32. Several doctoral studies have contributed to our understanding of ethics and morals in nursing. We can note only a few examples. Catherine Murphy, "Levels of Moral Reasoning in a Selected Group of Practitioners," Teachers College, Columbia University, 1976. Patricia Munhall, "Moral Reasoning Levels of Nursing Students and Faculty in a Baccalaureate Nursing Program," Teachers College, 1979. E.O. Bridston. Sarah T. Fry.

33. Kohlberg, op. cit.

34. D.E. Reilly, *Teaching and Evaluation the Affective Domain in Nursing Programs;* Thorofare, NJ: Slack, 1978. E.C. King, "Humanistic Education: Theory and Teaching Strategies," *Nurse Educator* 8, No. 4 (1983), 39–42. Id., *Affective Education in Nursing: A Guide to Teaching and Assessment;* Rockville, MD: Aspen, 1984.

This article is a longer version of one accepted for publication by *Nursing Outlook* during Fall 1988. Permission has been granted by Lucie Kelly, Editor, to use material in the published article within this volume.

CHAPTER 20

A CODE OF ETHICS FOR NURSE EDUCATORS

Marlene Merifield Rosenkoetter

[Rosenkoetter recognizes the growing interest in ethics for clinical nurses. Nurses who are teaching also need to be aware of the ethical dimensions of nursing education.]

During the past decade, interest in the impact of ethics and bioethics on nursing has increased. Ethical dilemmas in clinical practice and research and in the teaching of ethics have been emphasized, but the ethical problems of nurse educators have received little attention.

The existing codes of ethics of the American Nurses' Association and the International Council of Nurses, which were designed for the practicing clinical nurse, do not address many of the substantive ethical concerns of nursing faculty and educational administrators. My experience as a nursing faculty member and administrator has convinced me that ethical guidelines for education are needed. In 1981, I developed a preliminary code of ethics as part of a presentation on "Ethics in Nursing Education" at the annual meeting of the North Carolina League for Nursing. As a result of discussions of the code at that meeting and of a substantially revised code at the First International Congress on Nursing Law and Ethics held in Israel in 1982, the following code has been developed.

PREAMBLE

The Code of Ethics for Nurse Educators is based on the premise that each person involved in nursing education is unique and each has the right to have that uniqueness valued. The nurse educator functions as a teacher, clinician, researcher, mentor-counselor, and consultant and is responsible for adhering to ethical principles and established codes of ethics in each of these interrelated roles. The International Council of Nurses and the American Nurses' Association codes are considered basic codes for the practice of nursing and for nursing education.

Nurse educators have a responsibility for maintaining and promoting acceptable standards of nursing care and nursing education without discrimination with regard to race, color, religion, socioeconomic status, nationality, political affiliation, age, or sex. Nurse educators will:

[1] Assume responsibility and accountability for their actions in the practice of nursing and in the education of students.

[2] Function as advocates for students, clients, and faculty.

[3] Strive to promote critical thinking, effective decision making, caring, respect, and excellence in nursing.

[4] Facilitate and guide the learning of students in such a way as to reflect credit on nursing and nursing education.

[5] Equitably apply standards of performance to students and to themselves.

[6] Accept responsibility for contributing to the evolving body of nursing knowledge.

[7] Demonstrate respect for confidential matters relating to students, clients, and persons in the academic community.

[8] Accept the responsibility of maintaining their own competencies in nursing, in education, and in practice.

[9] Try to safeguard the client and the student from incompetent, illegal, or unethical practices by students, faculty, and other health care providers.

[10] Assume responsibility and accountability for their own practice of nursing.

[11] Deliberately limit their practice and teach within the scope of their own competencies.

[12] Participate in professional organizations, attesting to their commitment to the standards of nursing and to nursing education.

[13] Be accountable to students, to the academic community, to the profession and to society for fulfilling their academic responsibilities.

[14] Demonstrate respect for the rights of students regarding their participation in nursing research.

[15] Demonstrate respect for the student as a person and as an individual contributor to the profession and society.

REFERENCES

Marlene M. Rosenkoetter, "Ethics in Nursing Education," address, 29th annual meeting, North Carolina League for Nursing, Raleigh, NC, 20 Mar 81.

———, and, J. Rosenkoetter, "A Framework for Resolving Ethical Dilemmas in Nursing Education," pp. 151–159 in Nursing Law and Ethics ed. A. Carmi and S. Schneider; Berlin: Spring-Verlag, 1985.

The author extends appreciation to Alastair Campbell and Ingeborg Mauksch, participants in the First International Congress on Nursing Law and Ethics (Jerusalem, 1982), and other colleagues for their assistance in developing the code.

APPENDIX A

CODES OF ETHICAL BEHAVIOR

HIPPOCRATIC OATH

Codes of health care ethics are fairly ancient. One of the oldest is the well-known Hippocratic Oath. It dates officially from the Greek Hippocrates (460–377 B.C.), though more recent research credits much of it to the Cult of the Pythagoreans in the 4th century B.C. It has a stricter morality than that of Greek law or Platonic and Aristotelian ethics. It was not widely honored in the West until the Middle Ages. It may have influenced Indian traditions, known from a later time in the student's oath, "Charaka Samhita," c. 1 A.D. Both traditions put an emphasis on loyalty to the teacher and profession. Both put the patient's well-being above that of the practitioner.(1)

PERCIVAL'S CODE

A very influential code was that of Percival's *Medical Ethics* published in 1803 and republished by Chauncy Leake in 1927.(2) Thomas Percival's gentlemen's ethic was the basis of the Code adopted by the newly-formed American Medical Association in 1847. Percival followed the Hippocratic tradition. He urged physicians to keep their heads clear and their hands steady by observing the strictest temperance. His emphasis on professional etiquette was in marked contrast to the "quarrelsome conduct" of practitioners in that day. The AMA used the Code to exclude those not of their school, the so-called irregulars who had a new lease on life when Jacksonian democracy eliminated professional licensing laws. Increasingly from 1870 on, the Code was also used to eliminate Blacks and women from the physician role, an exclusion that the Flexner Report helped to near completion.(3)

FLORENCE NIGHTINGALE'S PLEDGE

Modern nursing stems from the work of Florence Nightingale (1820–1910), who focused on responsible obedience to the physician. The test came in the Crimean War (1854–1857), when the physicians would not allow the nurses on the battlefield, and she withheld her "troops" until the physicians were assured of that obedience. More recent research has stressed that she did not call for blind obedience. The Florence Nightingale Pledge long used in nursing says, "With loyalty will I endeavor to aid the physician in his work, and devote myself to the welfare of those committed to my care." Current emphasis is on intelligent obedience, as in the 1965 Code for Nurses of the International Council of Nurses (ICN).

ANA AND ICN CODES

The concern for a code of ethics was present from the beginnings of the American Nurses' Association, but no formal code was promulgated until 1950. It was revised in 1976 and dropped the concept of obedience, as did the 1973 revision of the 1965 ICN Code. The ANA Code for Nurses speaks to collaborative relationships with members of the health professions and other citizens in order to meet the health needs of the public. The new emphasis is on professional responsibility and accountability. The ICN Code has a fourfold responsibility to promote health, to prevent illness, to restore health, and to alleviate suffering. The ANA Code has an expansion in its Interpretive Statements (1985). Ronald S. Gass notes the Code's "distinctiveness among codes of ethics." Though its form is hortatory, "The nurse provides . . .," "The nurse safeguards . . . ," "The nurse acts . . . ," it goes beyond prescriptive statements to advocate accountability to the client. The statements reflect an awareness of shifting roles and the complexity of modern health care. They identify the values and beliefs behind the ethical standards. There is a remarkable breadth of social and professional concern within the ANA Code for Nurses.(4)

One might compare the Code itself to the concept of morals as the "shoulds" and "oughts" of society, the normative or applied ethics of some interpreters. The Interpretive Statements might then be compared with our concept of ethics with its concern for reasons, e.g., "Each client has the moral right to determine what will be done with his/her person . . ." The Interpretive Statements were revised in 1985.

CONCLUSION

Ethical codes have proliferated among the many professions.(5) The variety is perhaps not as great as it seems, for many of the newer codes are modeled after others. The Canadian Nurses' Association follows the ICN Code, though the Order of Nurses of Quebec has developed its own and Province groups are developing their own.(6)

ENDNOTES

1. Hippocrates: The Theory and Practice of Medicine. NY: Philosophical Library, 1964. "Appendix. Section I. Oath of Hippocrates," EB 4:1731. D. Konold, "Codes of Medical Ethics. I. History," EB 1:162–171. L. Edelstein, "The Hippocratic Oath: Text, Translation and Interpretation," Bulletin of the History of Medicine, Suppl. 1 (1943), 1–64. Robert M. Veatch, "Codes of Medical Ethics. II. Ethical Analysis," EB 1:172–180. Arthur L. Basham, "Hinduism," EB 2:661–667.

2. Leake, Percival's Medical Ethics; Baltimore Williams & Wilkins, 1927.

3. J.C. Mohr, Abortion in America; NY: Oxford, 1978. A.M. Brandt, "The Ways and Means of American Medicine," HCR 13, No. 3 (June 83), 41–43. Paul Starr, The Social Transformation of American Medicine; NY: Basic, 1983, emphasizes the insecure profession's rise to power by limiting competition and giving their membership legitimacy.

4. EB 4:1789–1799.

5. R. Chalk, M.S. Frankel and S.B. Chafer, AAAS Professional Ethics Project: Professional Ethics Activities in the Scientific and Engineering Societies; Washington: AAAS, 1980.

6. Albert R. Jonsen, Arthur L. Jameton, and A. Lynch, "Medical Ethics, History of: North America in the Twentieth Century," EB 3:992–1004.

AMERICAN NURSES' ASSOCIATION CODE
FOR NURSES, 1976

1. The nurse provides services with respect for human dignity and the uniqueness of the client unrestricted by considerations of social or economic status, personal attributes, or the nature of the health problem.
2. The nurse safeguards the client's right to privacy by judiciously protecting information of a confidential nature.
3. The nurse acts to safeguard the client and the public when health care and safety are affected by the incompetent, unethical, or illegal practice of any person.
4. The nurse assumes responsibility and accountability for individual nursing judgments and actions.
5. The nurse maintains competence in nursing.
6. The nurse exercises informed judgment and uses individual competence and qualifications as criteria in seeking consultation, accepting responsibilities, and delegating nursing activities to others.
7. The nurse participates in activities that contribute to the ongoing development of the profession's body of knowledge.
8. The nurse participates in the profession's efforts to implement and improve standards of nursing.
9. The nurse participates in the profession's efforts to establish and maintain conditions of employment conducive to high-quality nursing care.
10. The nurse participates in the profession's efforts to protect the public from misinformation and misrepresentation and to maintain the integrity of nursing.
11. The nurse collaborates with members of the health professions and other citizens in promoting community and national efforts to meet the health needs of the public.

INTERNATIONAL COUNCIL OF NURSES
CODE FOR NURSES 1973:

ETHICAL CONCEPTS APPLIED TO NURSING

The fundamental responsibility of the nurse is fourfold: to promote health, to prevent illness, to restore health, and to alleviate suffering.

The need for nursing is universal. Inherent in nursing is respect for life, dignity, and rights of man. It is unrestricted by considerations of nationality, race, creed, color, age, sex, politics, or social status.

Nurses render health services to the individual, the family, and community and coordinate their services with those of related groups.

Nurses and People

The nurse's primary responsibility is to those people who require nursing care. The nurse, in providing care, promotes an environment in which the values, customs, and spiritual beliefs of the individual are respected.

The nurse holds in confidence personal information and uses judgment in sharing this information.

Nurses and Practice

The nurse carries personal responsibility for nursing practice and for maintaining competence by continual learning.

The nurse maintains the highest standards of nursing care possible within the reality of a specific situation.

The nurse uses judgment in relation to individual competence when accepting and delegating responsibilities.

The nurse when acting in a professional capacity should at all times maintain standards of personal conduct that reflect credit upon the profession.

Reprint by permission: International Council of Nurses, 3 Place Jean Marteau, 1201 Geneva, Switzerland.

Nurses and Society

The nurse shares with other citizens the responsibility for initiating and supporting action to meet the health and social needs of the public.

Nurses and Co-Workers

The nurse sustains a cooperative relationship with co-workers in nursing and other fields.

The nurse takes appropriate action to safeguard the individual when his care is endangered by a co-worker or any other person.

Nurses and the Profession

The nurse plays the major role in determining and implementing desirable standards of nursing practice and nursing education.

The nurse is active in developing a core of professional knowledge.

The nurse, acting through the professional organization, participates in establishing and maintaining equitable social and economic working conditions in nursing.

AMERICAN MEDICAL ASSOCIATION PRINCIPLES OF MEDICAL ETHICS (1980)

PREAMBLE

The medical profession has long subscribed to a body of ethical statements developed primarily for the benefit of the patient. As a member of this profession, a physician must recognize responsibility not only to patients, but also to society, to other health professionals, and to self. The following Principles adopted by the AMA are not laws, but standards of conduct which define the essentials of honorable behavior for the physician.

(I)

A physician shall be dedicated to providing competent medical service with compassion and respect for human dignity.

(II)

A physician shall deal honestly with patients and colleagues, and strive to expose those physicians deficient in character or competence, or who engage in fraud or deception.

(III)

A physician shall respect the law and also recognize a responsibility to seek changes in those requirements which are contrary to the best interests of the patient.

(IV)

A physician shall respect the rights of patients, of colleagues, and of other health professionals, and shall safeguard the patient confidences within the constraints of law.

(V)

A physician shall continue to study, apply, and advance scientific knowledge, make relevant information available to patients, colleagues, and

Principles of Medical Ethics of the AMA, 1980. Reprinted with permission of the American Medical Association.

the public, obtain consultation, and use the talents of other health professionals when indicated.

(VI)

A physician shall, in the provision of appropriate patient care, except in emergencies, be free to choose whom to serve, with whom to associate, and the environment in which to provide medical services.

(VII)

A physician shall recognize a responsibility to participate in activities contributing to an improved community.

SPOTLIGHT ON CONTRIBUTORS

Mila Ann Aroskar, associate professor in the School of Public Health, University of Minnesota, Ed.D., M.Ed., B.S.N., R.N., F.A.A.N., received her education at the College of Wooster, Columbia (M.Ed., 1968), and SUNY at Buffalo (Ed.D., 1976). She has specialized in public health nursing and ethics in health care. She has taught at SUNY (Buffalo) and at the University of Minnesota. She was a Joseph P. Kennedy Fellow in Medical Ethics, Harvard, and is a Fellow of the Hastings Center. She is co-author, with Anne J. Davis, *Ethical Dilemmas and Nursing Practice,* 2nd ed. (Norwalk, CT: Appleton-Century-Crofts, 1985).

Nora Kizer Bell, associate professor in and chair of the Philosophy Department, University of South Carolina, adjunct professor in USC's schools of Medicine and Public Health, resident ethicist in the USC School of Medicine, Ph.D., M.Ph., B.Sc., received her education at Randolph-Macon (Phi Beta Kappa, 1962), the University of South Carolina (M.Ph., 1969), and the University of North Carolina (Ph.D., 1978). Her dissertation was on "Ethical Considerations in the Allocation of Scarce Medical Resources." She has been a consultant to many hospitals in South Carolina and the southeast, works with community groups on AIDS, South Carolina Hospital Association's Committee on Aging and Long Term Care, South Carolina Medical Associations Ethics Committee, and South Carolina Bar Association's Committee on the Death with Dignity Act. Dr. Bell is a member of Omicron Delta Kappa, Golden Key National Honorary, was Outstanding Teacher of the Year at the University of South Carolina, Beaufort (1973), Mortar Board Woman of the Year, J. Marion Sims Award (1988) of the South Carolina Public Health Association, Mortar Board Excellence in Teaching Award (1988), EXXON Fellow in Ethics and Medicine at Baylor College of Medicine (1985). She edited *Who Decides? Conflicts of Rights in Health Care* (Clifton, NJ: Humana, 1982) and has published numerous articles on medical ethics and social and political philosophy.

Leah L. Curtin, editor (since 1979) of *Nursing Management* (formerly *Supervisor Nurse*), M.A., M.S., B.S., Diploma, received her education from Good Samaritan Hospital School of Nursing, the University of Cincinnati (B.S., 1976; M.S., 1977), Athenaeum of Ohio (M.A. in Philosophy, 1977) and did a clinical internship in ethics at the University Affiliated Cincinnati Center for Developmental Disabilities. She was associate editor *Nursing Management* for a year. Earlier she was an engineering assistant with AT&T and a staff nurse for several Cincinnati hospitals. She has been a consultant and lecturer in ethics since 1975 and has taught at Mount Saint Joseph, Children's Hospital Medical Center, University of Cincinnati, and Northern Kentucky University. She founded the National Center for Nursing Ethics and the Christian Family Center (Community Outreach Agency) in Cincinnati. She has also been editor of *Update on Ethics* and *The Journal of Nursing Ethics* and has served on a number of editorial and other boards and agencies. She holds a long list of honors and awards in paleontology, community service, and nursing. In addition to many articles and editorials, she has published four books including *Nursing Ethics: Theories and Pragmatics* with M. Josephine Flaherty (Bowie, MD: Brady, 1982). She has presented over 600 papers to various groups and attends thirty to fifty continuing education programs a year.

Anne J. Davis, professor of nursing at the University of California in San Francisco, Ph.D., D.Sc., M.S.N., B.S.N., F.A.A.N., received her education at Emory (B.S.N., 1955) in Atlanta, Georgia, Boston University (M.S.N.), and the University of California in Berkeley (Ph.D., 1968). She was a Kennedy Post-Doctoral Fellow in Ethics at Harvard. Emory awarded her an honorary D.Sc. and the American Nursing Association gave her their Human Rights Award in 1986. She is an elected Fellow of the American Academy of Nursing (F.A.A.N.) and of the Hastings Institute for Bioethics. She has authored numerous articles and several books, and writes a regular column in the *Western Journal of Nursing*.

Claire M. Fagin, dean (since 1977) of the School of Nursing at the University of Pennsylvania, Ph.D., D.Sc., M.A., B.S., received her education at Wagner (1948), Columbia (M.A., 1951), and New York University (Ph.D., 1964). She has received honorary D.Sc. from Lycoming College (1983), Cedar Crest College (1987), and the University of Rochester (1987). She has given serious attention to health policy issues related to nursing and to consumers' access to the health care system. She has worked as a staff nurse in Sea View Hospital on Staten Island and as a clinical instructor at Bellevue. She taught at NYU and Lehman where she chaired the Department of Nursing and was director of the Health Professions Institute at Montefiore. She has served on many boards, agencies, panels, and task forces on the state, federal, and international levels and on several editorial boards of journals. She received the Founder's Award from Sigma Theta Tau in 1981, one of the first two Distinguished Scholar's Awards of the American Nursing Foundation in 1984, the American Psychiatric Nurses' Association & Journal of Psychosocial Nursing Award (1988), and the first Honorary Recognition Award of the American Nurses Association in 1988. She is a member of the Institute of Medicine, National Academy of Sciences, and American Academy of Nursing. She was president of the American Orthopsychiatric Association, 1985–86. She has published *Readings in Child and Adolescent Psychiatric Nursing* (1974), *Physical Assessment Lecture Series* (1974), and numerous articles and is a frequent speaker on radio and television.

Marsha Diane Mary Fowler, associate professor of Nursing and Theology at Azusa Pacific University, Ph.D., M.S., B.S., R.N., was educated at the Kaiser Foundation School of Nursing (1969), University of California, San Francisco (B.S., M.S.), and the University of Southern California at Los Angeles (Ph.D., 1984) and Harvard University. She has specialized in respiratory clinical nursing and ethics. She has taught at the University of Southern California at Los Angeles, Harvard University, and California State University at Los Angeles. She was a Joseph P. Kennedy Jr. Fellow in Medical Ethics (Harvard University), held the California Thoracic Society Teaching Fellowship, and received the University of Southern California President's Circle Scholarship. She is the author of numerous publications.

Sara T. Fry, associate professor at the University of Maryland School of Nursing, Baltimore (philosophy of nursing science and nursing ethics), Ph.D., M.S., B.S.N., R.N., received her education from The Johns Hopkins Hospital School of Nursing (Diploma in Nursing), the College of Nursing, University of South Carolina at Columbia (B.S.N.), the University of North Carolina at Chapel Hill (M.S. in public health nursing education), and Georgetown University (Ph.D. in philosophy with a focus on bioethics). Dr. Fry practiced nursing for over thirteen years in acute care and public health settings. She was a Kennedy Fellow in Medical Ethics at Georgetown, 1981–82, and has received several honors and awards for her work in bioethics. Dr. Fry has also taught in the School of Nursing, University of Virginia. She is the past chair of the Forum on Bioethics, American Public Health Association, and is current chair of the Committee on Ethics, Virginia Nurses' Association. She is a peer reviewer for several professional journals, a contributing editor for nursing journals, and has published and presented numerous papers, nationally and internationally, on bioethics, health care technologies, and moral accountability in nursing practice. She is the co-author with Robert M. Veatch of *Case Studies in Nursing Ethics* (Philadelphia: Lippincott, 1987).

Richard Thompson Hull, associate professor in philosophy and clinical assistant professor in the School of Medicine and a member of the graduate faculty at the State University of New York in Buffalo (where he has taught since 1967, Ph.D., B.A., received his education at Park College, Oklahoma City University, Austin College (in Sherman, Texas; B.A. in philosophy, 1963), and Indiana University (Ph.D. in philosophy, 1971). He has taught at Indiana and SUNY. He has also been headmaster of Calasanctius Preparatory School in Buffalo. The recipient of numerous grants and awards, he has published widely. Among his works are series of essays on nursing ethics and on medical ethics. The two essays published in this volume are part of a series done for the *Kansas Nurse* while he was in Houston, Texas, in personnel work which involved placement for nurses and other health care professionals. The series arose out of interviews with employers and employees about job stability. Hull is a member in the American Philosophical Association, Hastings Center, American Society for Value Inquiry (past president), Society for the Philosophy of Sex and Love, United University Professions/American Federation of Teachers, and served on the Committee for the Scientific Investigation of Claims of the Paranormal.

Myra Estrin Levine, professor of nursing at the University of Chicago, M.S.N., B.S., received her education at the Cook County (Chicago) School of Nursing (1944), the University of Chicago (B.S., 1949) and Wayne State University in Detroit (M.S.N., 1962). She has also taught at Loyola University in Chicago, the University of Illinois Health Science Center (adjunct professor of humanistic studies), Tel Aviv University and Ben Gurion University of the Negev in Israel (visiting professor), and Cook County School of Nursing. She served as administrative supervisor for the Henry Ford Hospital. She is a fellow in the American Academy of Nursing (charter member) and belongs to the American Nursing Association, Sigma Theta Tau, and the Oncology Nursing Society. She was the first recipient of the Elizabeth Russell Belford Award for Excellence in Teaching, honorary recognition from the Illinois Nursing Association. Her publications include *Introduction to Clinical Nursing; Renewal for Nursing; Four Conservation Principles of Nursing;* and over fifty articles.

Kathleen A. Mahon, Ed.D., M.S.N., B.S.N., A.A.N., received her education from San Francisco Community College (A.A.N., 1967) and from the University of California in San Francisco (B.S.N., 1972; M.S.N., 1973; and Ed.D., 1981). She has been a staff nurse (medical-surgical, Seton Medical Center, Daley City; maternal-child health and coronary care, Kaiser Permanente, San Francisco and San Rafael) and coordinator of perinatal services (Burlingame, California). She has served as a clinical evaluator (New York Regents College) and consultant (in education and with both state and federal governments) and has taught in the School of Nursing, University of San Francisco and DeAnza Community College (Cupertina). She was a postgraduate Fellow in Medical Ethics at Harvard (1978). In addition to extensive contributions in ethics, her research has included comparable worth and classification, civil rights, stress testing, and nursing curricula. She is active in the Peninsula Association for Retarded Children and Adults, working in education and housing.

Rita J. Payton, professor of nursing and director of the School of Nursing, University of Tulsa, Oklahoma, D.A., M.S., B.S., received her education from St. Mary's (Notre Dame, Indiana; B.S., 1960), Indiana (M.S., 1961), the University of North Colorado (D.A. in bioethics education, 1978). She taught for almost twenty years at the University of North Colorada in Greeley and earlier served as a staff nurse and instructor. She holds honors from Kappa delta Pi, Pi Lambda Theta, and Sigma Theta Tau, and was a Kennedy Foundation Fellow in Bioethics. Dr. Payton belongs to the American Nurses Association (Ethics Committee, 1976–82), National League of Nursing, the Hastings Center, and serves on a number of health care and other service groups. She has published many papers and several audiocassettes and is a nationally known public speaker and consultant.

Marlene Merifield Rosenkoetter, dean of the School of Nursing, University of North Carolina (Wilmington), Ph.D., M.S.N., M.Ed., B.A., received her education in Barnes Hospital School of Nursing (1964), University of Missouri (B.A., 1970; M.Ed., 1972), St. Louis University (Ph.D., 1979), and East Carolina University (M.S.N., 1983). She has specialized in community and mental health, and curriculum research. She has taught at Western Piedmont, Morganton, and the University of North Carolina (Wilmington) where she chaired the Department of Nursing. The author of numerous articles, she is a national and international consultant and active in many nursing associations.

Sharon Jeanne Smith, the College of Santa Fe, New Mexico, Ph.D., M.S., received her education from Boston College, (B.S.N.), University of California in San Francisco (M.S. in adult psychiatric nursing), and the Graduate Theological Union in Berkeley (Ph.D. in epistemology and ethics). She created the staff development office in psychiatric nursing in the Oakland Community Hospital and worked with staff nurses in ethics and patient care. At the University of California in San Francisco, she collaborated with Anne J. Davis on the article included in this volume.

Henry O. Thompson, adjunct professor of ethics in the School of Nursing, University of Pennsylvania and professor of Bible and ministry at the Unification Theological Seminary, Ph.D., M.A., M.Sc., B.Sc., Diploma, received his education at Iowa State University (B.Sc., 1953), Drew University (M.Div., 1958; Ph.D., 1964), Syracuse University (M.Sc. in education, 1971), Jersey City State College (M.A. in education psychology, 1975; Diploma in School Psychology, 1976) and Rutgers University (Newark, 24 hours). In addition to pastoral counseling and psychology, he has worked in biblical studies, archaeology, and ethics. He has served a number of churches in Minnesota and New Jersey. Dr. Thompson has taught in Upsala College, Colgate-Rochester Divinity School, New York Theological Seminary, University of Jordan, Jersey City State College, and Eastern College. He has authored and co-authored, edited and co-edited twenty books and has published numerous articles, reviews, and newspaper essays.

Joyce E. Beebe Thompson, professor and director of the graduate program in nurse-midwifery at the University of Pennsylvania, Dr. P.H., C.N.M., F.A.A.N., received her education at the University of Michigan (B.S.N., M.P.H.), the Maternity Center Association School of Nurse-Midwifery, and Columbia University (Dr.P.H.). She was a medical missionary in Chile for the United Methodist Church, and has taught at the State University of New York—Downstate (Brooklyn), Columbia University, and the University of Pennsylvania. She has specialized in nurse-midwifery and ethics. She chaired the American College of Nurse-Midwifery Division of Examiners for twelve years and served as ACNM president (1989). She has published, with Henry O. Thompson, *Ethics in Nursing* (NY: Macmillan, 1981), *Bioethical Decision Making for Nurses* (Norwalk, CT: Appleton-Century-Crofts, 1985), and numerous articles.

Robert M. Veatch, professor of medical ethics in the Kennedy Institute of Ethics, Georgetown University, professor of philosophy at Georgetown (since 1981), and adjunct professor in the departments of Community and Family Medicine and in Obstetrics and Gynecology in the

School of Medicine (since 1984), Ph.D., M.S., B.D., B.S., received his education at Purdue (B.S. *summa cum laude* in pharmacology, 1961), the University of California Medical Center in San Francisco (M.S. in pharmacology, 1962) and Harvard University (B.D. *magna cum laude,* 1967; M.A., 1970; Ph.D. in medical ethics, 1971). He taught at the University of Ife in Ibadan and high school in Ogbomosho in Nigeria, at Harvard University and Columbia University, and then was on the staff of the Hastings Center—The Institute of Society, Ethics, and the Life Science in Hastings-on-Hudson, New York (1970–79). He has also taught at Brown, Dartmouth, Manhattanville, Vassar, and the New School. A consultant and member of important boards and organizations, Dr. Veatch is well known for his many writings. In addition to hundreds of articles, among his many books are *Death, Dying and the Biological Revolution* (1976), *Value-Freedom in Science and Technology* (1976), *Case Studies in Medical Ethics* (1977), *A Theory of Medical Ethics* (1981), and co-authored with Sarah Fry, *Case Studies in Nursing* (1987).

SOURCES

WWAN = Jeffrey Franz, ed., *Who's Who in American Nursing;* Washington, D.C.: Society of Nursing Professionals, 1984; 2nd ed, 1987. *Who's Who in American Women,* 15th ed; Wilmette, IL: Marquis' *Who's Who,* 1988.

INDEX